THE
WAY
WE DIE

Brain death,
vegetative state,
euthanasia and other
end-of-life dilemmas

D1280188

THE
WAY
WE DIE

Brain death, vegetative state, euthanasia and other end-of-life dilemmas

---

LESLIE IVAN
with contributions by
MAUREEN MELROSE

Pari
Publishing

PARI PUBLISHING

Leslie Ivan MD, FRCSC, FACS, former head of neurosurgery at the Children's Hospital of Eastern Ontario, and Chair of the Division of Neurosurgery, University of Ottawa is now Emeritus Professor at the Faculty of Medicine, University of Ottawa. He is the author of 18 chapters, co-author and co-editor of three medical books. Among his numerous publications several papers and chapters deal with brain death, vegetative state and transplantation. He was among the first, in 1973, to describe and classify spinal reflexes in brain death.

Before coming to Canada in 1957, he was the Chief of Neurosurgery in one of the largest hospitals in Budapest but after the fall of the Hungarian revolution, he had to leave his homeland. He immigrated to Canada in 1957 and since 1967 he has been living in Ottawa. In 1995, he received the Kalman Santha Memorial Plaque and the Freedom Fighter's Medal and in 2006, on the fiftieth anniversary of the Hungarian revolution, the order of the Hungarian Republic's Officer's Crest.

Maureen Melrose RN (ret.d), was born in Saskatchewan, Canada where she completed her nurses' training. She worked in the operating room for several years where she and Leslie were destined to meet. Nursing was set aside for a time because of the needs of their family until it became possible to update her nursing skills. It was during this time that Maureen became interested in the ways to meet the needs of those patients and their relatives who were confronting the dilemmas associated with death. She gained valuable insights into their fears and needs and constantly looked for ways to ease their suffering and worry.

Maureen has had many interests. She trained as a musician and worked in the travel industry for ten years. But it was after a course in journalism at Carleton University that she began to work with Leslie on his many and varied writing projects. She has collaborated with her husband for many years as an editor and co-author.

Leslie and Maureen have been happily married for forty-four years, raised six children and have eleven grandchildren.

"Dr. Leslie Ivan and Maureen Melrose have written a wonderfully lucid and comprehensive account covering many important aspects dealing with death and dying. A discussion of brain death serves as a foundation for later considerations that deal with the hospice/palliative care movement, organ transplantation, the vegetative state, and physician-assisted suicide/euthanasia or death-hastening measures. The text is beautifully written, rooted in the best available evidence, evenly balanced in the opinions expressed, extensively referenced and infused with humanism and compassion. Highly recommended for both the interested layperson and professional health care worker."

John F. Seely, MD, PhD, FRCPC,
Palliative Care Consultant, Ottawa Hospital
Emeritus Professor and former Dean, Faculty of Medicine, University of Ottawa.

"*The Way We Die* is an important contribution to dialogue concerning the end of life in the human body. The Ivans have built a fair and broad understanding of various ethical approaches to the right-to-life and euthanasia discussion, but its use does not end there. The discussion of when death occurs and what happens to the body, persona, psyche, mind and even the soul sets a foundational understanding which can bring care workers in the hospital and hospice setting together.

This book is a must read for all palliative care workers, lay and professional. *The Way We Die* can add meaning and depth to the training of paramedics, doctors and nurses (and hospital administrators!), through its careful and respectful approach to faith-based assumptions about death. It ought to be the center of many discussion groups and book clubs, in churches and neighbourhoods! Well written, understandable language and logic contribute to making this book a "keeper" which sits on my bookshelf beside Kübler-Ross and Becker; a reminder of the pathway forward in a tangled area of ethical thought."

Rev. Brian S. Kopke, Minister Emeritus, First Unitarian Congregation of Ottawa
Past member of the Thomas Jefferson University Hospital Medical Ethics Committee, Philadelphia, Pennsylvania
Past Chair of the Medical Ethical Committee of the Regional Municipality of Ottawa Carleton, Ontario, Canada.

"This book is authoritative, comprehensive, and erudite. The authors lucidly take one through the development of many concepts which relate to dying—the concept of 'brain death', incognitive states and comas, palliative care, living wills and advance directives, euthanasia, and the philosophy of the mind, body and soul—as these concepts have evolved over a period of changing technology.

It will be of help to those who face end-of-life situations, such as palliative-care physicians and intensivists, neurosurgeons and neurologists, bereavement counselors, pastoral care persons, lawyers, ethicists and philosophers.

The ethical dilemmas are clearly laid out without drawing unjustifiable conclusions, and those who wish to enlighten themselves in all aspects of this difficult subject will find illumination here."

John B. Dossetor, OC, BM, BCh (Oxon.), FRCPC, PhD, Emeritus Professor (Medicine, Bioethics),University of Alberta, Canada, former internist and transplant nephrologist.

"The best overview I have read on the topic, incorporating history, various perspectives and the common sense of a clinician who has first hand insight into this delicate field. Extremely well written and concise and should serve as standard reading in medical school curricula. Even more so, it should be a standard reference for anyone who still agonizes about the brain death concept, life, death and technology. A vital piece of work. It was a pleasure to read and comforting to know that others in medicine consider/deliberate /pensively articulate these issues. Bravo!"

Sam Shemie, MD, Division of Pediatric Critical Care, Medical Director, Extracorporeal Life Support Program, Montreal Children's Hospital, McGill University Health Centre. Associate Professor of Pediatrics, McGill University.

"Leslie Ivan is an experienced clinician as well as a brilliant writer. He is the ideal person to present the latest information on medical advances about death and dying in this fascinating and easy to read book. We learn that human life does not end with a "sudden lightning", but mostly as a process. If you are facing a medical or ethical end-of-life dilemma, or if you are just interested in objective up-to date information about death and dying, this is your book."

Johannes Kuchta, MD, Department of Neurosurgery, University Hospital, University of Cologne, Germany. Member of the European Brain and Behaviour Society (EBBS).

ISBN 978-88-901960-3-4

Book design and cover by Andrea Barbieri
Cover photo © Fedor Sidorov - Fotolia

Pari Publishing

Via Tozzi 7, 58040 Pari, Grosseto, Italy
www.paripublishing.com

Thoughts and dedications

To our children: Agnes, Andrea, Patricia, Christopher and Jennifer
and the memory of Judy

"What I have to say has all been said before,
And I am destitute of learning and of skill with words,
I therefore have no thoughts that this might be of benefit to others
I wrote it only to sustain my understanding."

Shantideva (AD 687-763)

Table of Contents

Prologue **17**

Preface **19**

Introduction and Acknowledgments **21**

CHAPTER 1 **THE ROAD TO THE CONCEPT OF BRAIN DEATH** **25**

Death as a biological process 25

The death of cells 26

The death of organs 27

A short history of the determination of death 28

From consciousness to coma 31

Consciousness 31

Coma 34

Coma and brain resuscitation 39

The diagnosis and management of coma 42

CHAPTER 2 **BRAIN DEATH** **49**

Evolution of the concept 49

An acceptable definition 53

Medical limitations 54

Controversies about the time of death 56

The law and the criteria of death 60

Irreversible coma and brain death 61

Brain death worldwide 65

CHAPTER 3 **OTHER ISSUES RELATED TO DEATH**.. **73**

Dying with Dignity 73

The hospice concept and palliative care 74

The "right to die" movement and assisted suicide 77

The patient's rights 78

The doctor's obligation.. 81

The "Do not resuscitate" order 83

The Living Will... 86

CHAPTER 4 **ORGAN TRANSPLANTATION AND THE TIME SEQUENCE IN BRAIN DEATH....... 91**

Organ donation and transplantation protocols............... 98

CMA policy statement about transplantation................. 104

CHAPTER 5 **THE VEGETATIVE STATE 109**

Definition.. 110

Historical evolution of the term and prevalence of the condition 111

Neuropathology 112

Diagnosis of the vegetative state............................... 113

The natural course of PVS... 115

Well known cases of vegetative state.......................... 117

CHAPTER 6 **EUTHANASIA.............................. 133**

Definition.. 133

The roots and growth of the pro-euthanasia movement .. 135

The ethical roots of anti-euthanasia............................ 137

Euthanasia and the law... 140

Euthanasia and public opinion 146

The future of assisted death 148

CHAPTER 7 **LIFE AFTER DEATH**...................... **157**
Our concern with life after death 157
The near-death experience 160
The problem of mind, body and soul........................... 165

Journals and abbreviations **175**

Glossary of terms.. **179**
Books 189
Journals.. 194
Internet resources 201

Appendix A.. **207**
World Medical Association Declaration on Death.......... 207

Appendix B **209**
Diagnosis of Death in U. K. 209

Appendix C... **213**
Guidelines for the Diagnosis of Brain Death 213

Appendix D **223**
Uniform Determination of Death Act, USA 223

Appendix E **227**
Euthanasia and assisted suicide (update 1998)...... 227

Prologue

It is a particular pleasure to write this prologue since in doing so it evokes for me fond memories of the many times I have sat in the Ivans' home and discussed–among many other topics–the ethical, legal and moral dilemmas a neurosurgeon encounters in professional life–issues that are so clearly explained in the present book.

My first encounter with Leslie Ivan was after receiving a telephone call from the emergency wing of the Children's Hospital of Eastern Ontario. It was there that I learned that my son Jason had been involved in an accident with a golf club, which had fractured his forehead and driven some of the bone into the front of his brain. Ivan's first words to me were that I should focus on the fact that my son was still alive, and keep this at the front of my mind. He then transferred Jason to the operating room.

Following the emergency surgery, and after several days of sedation, Jason's first act was to paint a large, yellow "happy face", which the staff displayed at one of the hospital windows. We knew then that the prognosis was to be a good one. And, who knows, maybe something rubbed off from Leslie Ivan in that operating room, for many years later Jason worked in Africa, Indonesia and Afghanistan for Médecins Sans Frontières, and is now working with the Canadian Red Cross on their Malaria Project for Africa.

My own experience was one out of the countless number of incidents in which relatives must face the consequences of head injury—the possibility of brain damage and even the death of their loved ones. At one time we human beings identified ourselves with the heart, but today we know that the organ of personality, memory and will resides in the brain and, even if the phenomenon of consciousness is still being endlessly debated by philosophers and neuroscientists, at least we agree that when that organ dies then personality disappears from earth. Yet, as the present book explains, in so many cases there is no simple either/or condition involved but a variety of levels that can be medically assessed. These can range from temporary coma to a persistent vegetative state, or from the bizarre "locked-in state" in which higher brain function persists yet with a compromised brainstem, to states of true "brain death" where the physical structure of the cortex and neocortex has been irreversibly destroyed.

In each of these cases there are legal, ethical and moral decisions to be made and it is here that doctors seek the help of their professional organizations, legal institutions and religious leaders. Those were the sorts of issues that I would discuss with Maureen and Leslie Ivan over a glass of wine late into the evening. It is a true pleasure for me to relive them by reading the present book with all its depth, compassion and precision of exposition.

F. David Peat, PhD
Author and Director of the Pari Center for New Learning

Preface

The cultural anthropologist, Ernest Becker, in his 1973 Pulitzer Prize-winning book, *Denial of Death*, has posed that the fear of death is the predominant fear in man and that we cope with this fear by denying its inevitability. We push it out of mind by filling our mind and days with busyness and activity. Death has been a taboo subject. This leads to a striking lack of knowledge of death and the dying process. However in the past few decades one could not have avoided being aware of all the emotional, social, legal and ethical aspects of dying and conditions that approach death.

One of the best ways of overcoming fear is knowledge of that which we most fear. This book by the husband and wife team of neurosurgeon Dr. Leslie Ivan and Maureen Melrose Ivan, RN, goes a long way towards explaining the biological basis for the dying process and in particular the relatively recent concept of brain death. The brain is also subject to a number of conditions that result from varying degrees of structural and functional damage. Some of these, such as persistent vegetative state, have, with some justification, been considered as worse than death. Medical scientific advances in the past few decades have enabled physicians to sustain patients with previously fatal organ failure to survive almost indefinitely.

Along with these technical blessings have come extremely difficult problems of ethics and law that tax our levels of compassion. The Ivans discuss these various aspects of medical care, drawing on their many years of experience in which they have shown both technical skill and inspiring humanism. Though undoubtedly having personal convictions they have not let them interfere with presenting a wide range of opinion in these many thorny issues. The book is well referenced, almost encyclopedic, and covers almost every related issue, including even near-death experiences and assisted suicide.

This book is clearly written so that it can be read and appreciated by the general public yet still provide information and useful reference for even the most experienced care givers. *The Way We Die* is one of the most informative writings on the subject and the information presented will go a long way toward the understanding dying and dispel much of the innate fear of death and dying that haunts all of us.

Robert F. Nelson, BSc, MD, FRCP(C)
Former Professor and Head, Division of Neurology,
University of Ottawa,
Former Chair, Clinical Ethics, The Ottawa Hospital.

Introduction and Acknowledgments

What is not fully understood is not possessed
Johann Wolfgang von Goethe

No matter when or how we die, adult or child, it is and always has been the death of the brain that made the dying process irreversible. For many hundreds of years cessation of heartbeat and respiration as markers of life's end were never challenged until the discovery, in the 18th century, that some people could be revived from apparent death. Yet, it wasn't until two centuries later, in the mid nineteen fifties that medical technology had advanced enough for us to understand that death occurs in stages and that the stage of irreversibility coincides with the death of the brain.

As a medical and legal definition, brain death has been widely accepted though it is still, on occasion, misunderstood and, in fact, has created certain end-of-life dilemmas, disagreements and contention. Certain issues, especially those related to the vegetative state and assisted dying have been widely debated in science, ethics, religion and the law.

This is why, in the first two chapters of the book, we explore consciousness and the stages of coma and brain death to lay the foundation for a discussion of the vegetative state, euthanasia, the near-death experience, and other related, contentious issues. The exploration of brain death lends itself to the consideration of organ donation. We discuss transplantation protocols and show statistical figures from the United Kingdom and the United States to highlight the importance of transplantation surgery and organ donation. We describe how the removal of organs is practiced today to satisfy ethical and legal requirements to sustain life for the benefit of thousands of patients.

A respect for life should involve respect for the wishes of a dying person. We feel that as a humanistic duty and an expression of our love for another human being, the fear and pain of death should be alleviated as much as possible. There are choices that a dying patient may have made in advance verbally or in writing about administration or cessation of certain treatments. We have included information about the Living Will or other advanced directives and about palliative care and its many benefits without excluding the pros and cons of euthanasia.

Even with little medical knowledge readers should be able to understand almost everything in this book; nevertheless, there is a glossary of terms for those who need assistance. We have tried to make the text as easy to read as possible and have added a significant number of references for further study. The bibliography has been compiled for those who wish to find related material in medical, legal, religious and philosophical books and relevant publications, including those on the Internet. Additional reading may provide the reader with a deeper understanding of all issues, and the ever-changing concerns and controversies. Associated professionals, not only in medicine, but in the fields of religion, ethics and the law, could find some of the facts and ideas in the book useful.

Researching and writing this book would not have been possible without the contribution of many people; friends, colleagues, artists and librarians. First we should acknowledge the immense help we have received from Dr. Robert Nelson, who carefully read the manuscript. He kindly suggested certain changes and wrote his thoughtful preface. We owe words of gratitude to a number of libraries that helped us to find much-needed material: The Health Science Library at the University of Ottawa, the Public Library of Ottawa's Elmvale Branch and the Greater Victoria Public Library's Main Branch.

We owe our gratitude and thanks for permission to reproduce copyrighted material from the following sources: The Canadian Medical Association and its CMA Journal, the Canadian Journal of Neurological Sciences, the British Medical Journal, the Toronto University Press and Irwin Law Publisher. Our special thanks are due to Trevor Jones at UK Transplant for his personal help with statistical figures, and to Dr. Johannes Kuchta, neurosurgeon (Department of Neurosurgery, University of Cologne) who, in addition to providing copyrighted material, helped us with his excellent Power Point presentation and other references on brain death. Our gratitude goes to Ros Salvador who provided much-needed help with the latest legal status of brain death legislation in Canada and to John M. McCabe, Legislative Director of the National Conference of Commissioners on Uniform State Laws in the United States for his permission to reprint the Uniform Determination of Death Act.

We would like to express our most sincere thanks to a number of highly esteemed professors, colleagues and friends, who had read and commented on the manuscript or the galley proofs. In Ottawa, Senator Wilbert Keon, Professors John Dossetor and John Seely, Reverend Brian Kopke and in Montreal Professor Sam Shemie, all of whom, despite their heavy professional commitments, graciously read the galley proofs.

We are grateful to Emil Purgina, an old friend and artist, who did the illustrations and to Andrea Barbieri for a beautiful book design. Special thanks to Eleanor Peat at Pari Publishing for her continuing interest and help and to Maureen Doolan for her superbly constructive, meticulous and innovative editing which not only improved the text, but made cooperation and communication easy for us. Happily, we also located David Peat, a writer friend and educator, whom we have known since his Ottawa days, and would like to thank him for a warm and cordial prologue.

As authors, we are very grateful to have been able to work together for so many years. We wrote this book because we believe that a more complete understanding of death and dying will enable people to face end-of-life dilemmas, should they arise, with calmness, knowledge, understanding and compassion.

Leslie Ivan and Maureen Melrose
Ottawa, February 2007

CHAPTER 1
THE ROAD TO THE CONCEPT OF BRAIN DEATH

The concept and verification of death has undergone many changes during the millennia of human existence. The latest change, a paradigm shift, was brought about by the success of **resuscitation*** technology in the middle of the twentieth century. Despite saving many lives, resuscitation efforts often failed and "**beating heart cadavers**", oxygenated by a **mechanical respirator**, started to occupy the essential beds in Intensive Care Units.

In order to fully understand this new concept of death, it might be helpful to explore death from several angles before we move to discuss **brain death** itself and other end-of-life dilemmas that in a few decades have polarized legal and ethical thought and public opinion.

Death as a biological process

Death is an entity common to all living organisms in the earth's biosphere. Since the cell is the basic unit of all living organisms, to take into account the interesting way cells die might be a good way to approach the death of organs, which in turn, should ease the comprehension of how the human brain dies.

---

* *Definitions of terms in bold type are listed in the Glossary on page 179*

The death of cells

Textbooks of pathology describe cell death as **necrosis**. Necrosis (in Greek nekros=dead) is the death of a circumscribed area of animal tissue as a result of an outside agent and may follow a wide variety of injuries, both physical (cuts, burns, bruises) and biological (effects of disease-causing agents). The morphological appearance of necrotic tissue in any organ can be detected by the naked eye and the damaged or destroyed cells have characteristic changes that reveal the stages of death of cell groups when tissues are examined under the microscope. Among the environmental perturbations that may cause cell necrosis are oxygen deprivation (**anoxia**), **hypothermia**, immunological attack and exposure to various toxins that inhibit crucial intracellular metabolic processes.

But cells may die by design as well as by accident. Research in developmental pathology refers to this as programmed cell death. In vertebrates it has been called **apoptosis** and in invertebrates, cell deletion. Such programmed events are essential if the organism as a whole is to develop its normal final form. Waves of genetically driven cell death are critical to the proper modelling of organs and systems.

Programmed cell death may also play a part in the process of aging, cells being designed to die after a certain number of **mitotic** divisions. Groups of cells responsible for the color of human hair, for instance, may cease to function years before the hair itself loses the capacity to grow: the result is the "uncolored" white hair of old age.

The cells in human beings, all thirty trillion of them, are united and coordinated by the most complex organizational system known today. The death of single cells is a progressive phenomenon, a microscopic counterpart of the death of the higher organism. Studies have shown that the moment of cell death is preordained and regulated by a relentless mechanism. Cells, after a certain life span which is characteristic for the cell type, become deficient in function before they die. This is the natural **senescence** of cells unless prematurely destroyed by trauma or disease. As certain cells die, others take their place and the dead cells provide the living cells with nourishment or information which regulates the organism. This regulation is quite astounding: in a normal adult, two hundred billion red cells die and are born every day! With the exception of nerve cells, all cells of the body are constantly being replaced, some more rapidly than others. (Veatch, 1989)[1] and (Hoffman, 1957).[2]

The two types of cell death, necrosis and apoptosis, have different morphological features. Furthermore, different intracellular mechanisms have been incriminated in their production. Necrosis, as in heart infarct (heart attack), occurs in a group of cells or in an entire organ, as in brain death. Necrosis is characterized by progressive changes from the moment of the insult until the whole organ loses all cellular elements and turns into dead tissue.

The death of organs

The organs of the human body (e.g. kidney, liver, brain) are differentiated structures consisting of cells and groups of cells distinctive to each organ that perform a specific function in the living organism. Some organs are so important that we cannot live without them because they are necessary for the maintenance of life (lungs, heart, brain, liver and kidneys for example), while others (the spleen, ovaries and testicles) are not important to sustain life. On the other hand, if there is only partial destruction of a vital organ, such as in cardiac **infarction** or the removal of one of the kidneys or lungs, normal living and reasonably good health can often be expected.

The integrity of the brain and its regulatory functions are necessary for life in higher organisms such as animals and human beings. Consequently, the viability of nerve cells and the life of an individual are vitally interdependent. Since the viability of nerve cells and the integrity of the brain depend on an uninterrupted oxygen supply, it follows that adequate respiration and circulation are essential not only for the brain but for the entire human body to survive. This is why the heart and the lungs are vital organs. They are vital because they ensure the survival of the nerve cells.

What about other vital organs? The kidneys and the liver are such examples. Both kidney and liver failure cause the accumulation of toxic chemicals that are harmful to the brain. These chemicals cause uremic (in the case of kidney failure) or hepatic (in the case of liver

failure) **encephalopathies** which are well known causes of **coma** and
death. As long as the brain is not damaged, **uremic** and **hepatic coma**
remains reversible.

With the exception of nerve cells, all cells of the body are constantly
replaced, some more rapidly than others. A cell is dead when it can
no longer maintain the specific composition which distinguishes it
from its environment. As cells die, organs can die and when vital
organs die, life can only be maintained artificially through kidney
dialysis, cardiac pacemakers, heart transplantation and **respirators**.
This process whereby "life" is restored or "death" is made reversible
is called resuscitation.

In the past, cardiorespiratory arrest or kidney or liver failure
would have meant death. Today, the use of modern chemical and
physical means and intensive care units replace missing regulatory
mechanisms and a transplant surgeon can replace missing organs so
that eternal prolongation of life appears almost feasible (Safar, 1978).[3]
But if you think more deeply about it, you will find that death must
remain a reality for the rest of the history of mankind. The limits of
resuscitation and the limits of transplant surgery are inherent in the
vulnerability of the nerve cells. Even though an individual may have
his heartbeat and respiration restored successfully (Ventureyra and
Ivan, 1979),[4] the amount of damage to the nerve cells will determine
the reversibility or finality of coma and death.

From a physiological point of view, the definition of death should
be "the permanent disappearance of every sign of life" as the United
Nations Vital Statistics states, or more clearly "the total cessation of
life processes that eventually occurs in all living organisms".

A short history of the
determination of death

Early human beings associated living with breathing and the earliest
recognition of death must have been the absence of respiration. For
thousands of years the cessation of life functions was determined

by the use of simple criteria. First it must have been the observation of a person who appeared to be sleeping but didn't breathe and couldn't be awakened by shouting or shaking the body. Then, in 1628 the discovery of the circulation of blood by William Harvey made heartbeat another obvious sign of life.[5] Thus, for the next three hundred years the absence of heartbeat and respiration was sufficient to establish that a person was dead.

It is quite remarkable how little knowledge was required for lay coroners to pronounce someone dead. However, because mistakes were made, it became common knowledge that death could be apparent rather than real and that seemingly dead persons could be revived. For the sake of reviving victims of drowning, asphyxiation and those who had been struck by lightning, the first Humane Society was established in Amsterdam in 1767. The idea was followed by the creation of the Royal Humane Society in London in 1774.[6] The movement soon reached North America and in 1780 the Philadelphia Humane Society was founded. These Societies, with the help of progressive physicians, had become involved in the re-examination of the traditional signs of death: absence of pulse and respiration, the observation of pallor, coldness and the stiffness of the body. All these signs could be present in victims of drowning yet revival was sometimes possible. The invention of the stethoscope in 1816 made it possible to add the absence of heart sounds as a further refinement to the criteria of death. Based on accumulating evidence that the reaction of the pupils to light was a sign of a potentially successful resuscitation, non-reactive pupils were added to the characteristic signs of death. *Black's Law Dictionary* (1951) defined death as: "total stoppage of the circulation of the blood and cessation of the animal and vital functions of the body such as respiration and pulsation".[7] *Dorland's Illustrated Medical Dictionary* in 1957 still defined death as: "the apparent extinction of life, as manifested by the absence of heartbeat and respiration".[8]

Death based on the above criteria, validated by a physician or a coroner, was rarely opposed by the law. However, the standard definitions had not anticipated the extensive use of cardiac massage, pacemakers, mechanical respirators and other modern resuscitation techniques. As Safar (1996) stated four decades later "the development of modern **cardiopulmonary-cerebral resuscitation (CPCR)** has given every person the ability to challenge death anywhere".[9]

These new advances in medical technology, that "revived" patients from the traditional definition of death, made "life" possible when neither heartbeat nor respiration was spontaneous. Yet, the resuscitated subject was, in some instances, totally unresponsive and exhibited the neurological characteristics of death: 1. absent **cephalic** reflexes, 2. absence of spontaneous respiration, and 3. no electrical activity from the **cerebral cortex**.

Aside from the outmoded legal definition of death, there were no legal or ethical guidelines for physicians on how to withdraw respiratory support when the brain appeared irreversibly damaged. Keeping victims of failed resuscitation in much needed beds in Intensive Care Units raised ethical questions of a different kind. It became apparent that without new criteria of death, hospitals would be filled with patients on respirators. Wards of active treatment would turn into weird pathological museums of bodies connected to breathing machines. The need for the concept of **"cerebral death"** developed, at least in part, from the imperatives of this Orwellian image about the future.

Finally, in 1957, the pressing problems forced French anesthesiologists to turn to Pope Pius XII for guidance concerning their ethical responsibilities to patients in deep coma whose respiration was maintained mechanically. A portion of the Pope's statement reads as follows:

> Since these forms of treatment go beyond the ordinary means to which one is bound, it cannot be held that there is an obligation to use them. . . . It remains for the doctor . . . to give a clear and precise definition of 'death' and the 'moment of death' of a patient who passes away in a state of unconsciousness.[10]

Among the first to describe this state of unconsciousness were French anesthetists (Mollaret and Goulon, 1959) who called this condition "le coma dépassé," a state beyond coma (or an irreversible coma).[11]

The ethical problems were augmented by the increasing need for kidney donations and the race for heart transplantation. To protect the interest of patients waiting desperately for donated organs, without compromising the chances for survival of those in a coma, committees were formed in hospitals and university centres to define new criteria of death.

The moral, ethical and legal aspects were particularly vexing for practising neurologists and neurosurgeons. Often they had to face the difficult question of how to manage their deeply comatose patients and to decide when their condition reached a point of no return. The greatest step towards a universally acceptable definition of irreversible coma was the establishment of the Ad Hoc Committee of Harvard Medical School in 1968 to examine the definition of brain death.[12]

From this definition the concept gradually evolved that the death of an individual could be equated with the death of his or her brain and that "cerebral death" could be diagnosed with reasonable certainty. This diagnosis required sophisticated equipment and trained minds rather than the traditional methods of inspection; **palpation** and **auscultation**.

To equate the death of a person with the death of the brain was a most momentous development in the history of medicine and mankind. The significance of these developments cannot be overestimated, since they influence individual morality, professional ethics, the law and, ultimately, the understanding of human beings, the relationship of mind, body and soul and, in turn, philosophy and religious thinking.

From consciousness to coma

Consciousness

John Locke, the English philosopher (1632-1704), defined consciousness as the perception of what passes in a man's own mind. It sounds so simple at first approach, but becomes more complicated when we ask a few relevant questions. What is the structure in our brain that generates this function we call consciousness? What are the characteristics of consciousness and of the loss of it? What is the difference between sleep, loss of consciousness and coma? How do we know that there is recovery from some forms of coma while at other times it is a state of no return? The answer to these questions depends on whom you ask and at what stage of our scientific knowledge.

Consciousness can be characterized and discussed from a variety of angles. The neurophysiologist (Adrian, 1964),[13] the biologist (Adam, 1980),[14] the psychobiologist (Davidson, 1980),[15] the neuropsychologist (Furst, 1979)[16] and the philosopher (Searle, 1997)[17] emphasise different aspects of this elusive function of the brain.

Consciousness, physiologists tell us, is the state of awareness of self and environment. Behavioral scientists would insist that consciousness is the behavioral manifestation of arousal and responsiveness to various stimuli. Psychiatrists talk about conscious and subconscious thoughts and acts, calling a thought or an act conscious when the individual knows that the thought or act is indeed happening. Clinically-oriented neuroscientists have been saying for decades that consciousness involves the sum of all cortical brain functions including memory, language, intelligence and particularly arousal, that is, the general excitatory effect of sensory stimulation resulting in alertness, vigilance and wakefulness.

The number of books examining consciousness from a philosophical point of view is quite extraordinary. These books are classified and listed by Flanagan (Flanagan, 1993).[18] He lists sixteen books in several categories (e.g. the phenomenology, the functional-computational, neuro-philosophical theories of consciousness) as the best collection of works on consciousness between 1972 and 1990. On the other hand, as Laurence O. McKinney (1994)[19] so aptly wrote about consciousness, "all forms of consciousness seem to require two parts of perception, the ability to extract useful information from the environment, and cognition, the manner in which that information triggers useful reaction. Limiting either limits our experience".

The finding of the anatomical substrate of arousal was one of the great leaps forward in understanding the "waking brain" in the 1950s.

Magoun,[20] a neurophysiologist, proved that the mechanisms responsible for arousal are in the core of the upper and lower brainstem and he called it the ascending reticular activating system (**ARAS**). The ARAS acts as an "on" and "off" switch that keeps the hemispheres of the brain awake (Fig. 1). Without the integrity of the arousal system (as is the case in irreversible coma), consciousness is not possible.

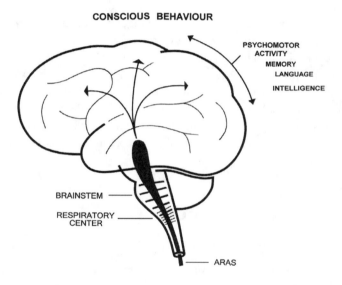

Fig. 1. *The diagram shows the left lateral surface of the brain with the cerebellum and the brainstem. The respiratory centre is in the lower brainstem (fine crosshatching). The ascending pathway of wakefulness, ARAS, ascending reticular activating system, (solid line), passes through the brainstem (crosshatched area) and projects through the higher brainstem to other parts of the brain. Conscious behavior is dependent on the interaction between the ARAS and the cerebral cortex.*

Before exploring further the nature of altered consciousness, we should discuss the difference between sleep and coma. Sleep is a normal, reversible state of decreased awareness and responsiveness, the opposite of wakefulness. But, unlike coma, one can be aroused from sleep because the arousal system is intact, whereas, in coma, either the arousal system (ARAS) is damaged or there is no neuronal network to be aroused in the higher brainstem or the cortex.

Sleep produces characteristic tracings on the **EEG (electro-encephalogram)**. The stages of sleep can be recognized and, with increasing depth of sleep, slower and slower wave forms will appear. These slow waves or delta waves of the EEG are very similar to the delta waves seen in coma except that, in deepening coma, arousal stimuli such as pain would not change the **delta activity**. With deepening coma the amplitude of the slow waves would gradually flatten until ultimately, all electrical activity might cease (Fig. 2).

The integrity of the nervous system and the maintenance of consciousness depend on a steady state, also called homeostasis of the intracranial contents. This homeostasis is dependent upon 1. a constant supply of oxygen, 2. a constant supply of glucose, 3. a constant elimination of metabolic wastes, and 4. maintenance of normal **intracranial pressure.**

Coma

Consciousness may be impaired by damage or injury to tissues or organs of the body that maintain this steady state. For example, lack of oxygen, as in suffocation; lack of glucose, as in **hypoglycemia**; insufficient elimination of metabolic wastes, as in kidney failure (uremia) or in liver disease (hepatic coma). All may impair consciousness due to interference with the normal function of the **neurons** (nerve cells) in the cerebral cortex or in the ARAS. As long as the neuronal damage is remediable, the coma itself remains reversible.

Coma becomes irreversible when nerve cells, both in the brainstem and in the cortex, are destroyed by lack of oxygen or by increased pressure inside the skull, as occurs following severe head injury and intracranial hemorrhage.

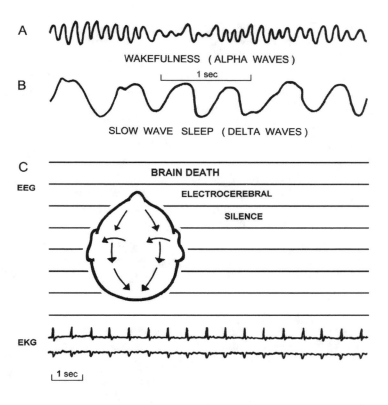

Fig. 2. *The illustration shows EEG wave forms characteristic for wakefulness, deep sleep and brain death.*
A. The type of waves we see in a wakeful, relaxed state, alpha waves: 8-12/sec. B. Slow wave activity in deep sleep, delta waves: 1.5-2/sec. C. Note the different time scale. This record was taken of a middle-aged female who suffered severe brain haemorrhage from a ruptured aneurysm. The brain damage was irreversible and ultimately ended in brain death. The EEG was recorded four days after the haemorrhage and shows "electrocerebral silence". The bottom two lines represent EKG recorded from the hands.

Increased intracranial pressure as a result of a brain tumor, hemorrhage or trauma will shift the brain downwards and compress the **midbrain** where the bulk of the ARAS is located. This is the commonest cause of deep coma in patients following a stroke or severe head injury. Depending on the degree of cell damage in the cortex or in the brainstem, the state of coma may or may not be reversible.

Coma, therefore, can be induced by two major mechanisms:

1. intracranial lesions (tumor, hemorrhage, infection, trauma), by virtue of abnormal pressure on the nerve cells in the cerebral cortex or in the brainstem. Increased intracranial pressure, the medical term for this condition, can be diagnosed clinically and measured with intracranial pressure monitors.
2. metabolic processes which interfere with normal functions of the nerve cells (e. g. uremia, diabetic coma, hypoglycemia, suffocation, drowning, drugs.)

According to the responsiveness of the nervous system, the alertness or the lack of it can be graded by certain clinical criteria. Tables I and II show two different systems of coma grading.

The Glasgow Coma Scale (GCS)[21] was first described by Teasdale and Jennett in the early 1970s. It has been the gold standard of neurological assessment of trauma patients since its development. The GCS is simple to use and it has been the method of choice to document neurologic findings over time and predict functional outcome in trauma care with brain injuries.

Table I

GLASGOW COMA SCALE

The grading system assigns numeric values to observed responses

Eye Opening	E	Best motor response	M	Verbal response	V
spontaneous	4	obeys commands	6	oriented	5
to speech	3	localizes	5	confused conversation	4
to pain	2	withdraws	4	inappropriate words	3
nil	1	abnormal flexion	3	incomprehensible sounds	2
		extends	2	nil	1
		nil	1		

EMV score or responsiveness sum between 3 and 15

If E+M+V score=13-15 (opens eyes, obeys commands and is verbally oriented) prognosis is favorable.

If E+M+V score=3-5 (no eye opening, abnormal motor or verbal response) the prognosis is poor.

For over thirty years the Glasgow Coma Score has been used more frequently than any other scale or method to describe impaired consciousness in emergency situations, particularly with head injures. Nevertheless, other systems have been developed (Lombardi, 2002)[22] and (Berger, 2001)[23] that have been tried either to refine GCS or compare it to other methods.

Table II

RESPONSIVENESS SCALE

The grading system depends on clinical description

Terms for decreased responsiveness	Clinical description
I Drowsiness	lethargic, somnolent, uninterested, easy to arouse, does not lapse into sleep immediately when left undisturbed
II Stupor	obtunded, disoriented, will lapse into sleep when undisturbed
III Deep stupor (semicomatose)	rouses on strong painful stimulus, may have focal neurological signs, motor responses are appropriate
IV Coma	does not respond appropriately, may have **decerebrate, decorticate** posturing, breathes spontaneously
V Deep coma	does not respond appropriately to any stimuli, limbs are flaccid, reflexes absent, may breathe spontaneously

These grading systems of disturbed consciousness serve as important guides to observe and treat a comatose patient. Along with the vital signs, the level of consciousness is carefully monitored at the bedside. A deepening coma is a powerful signal to use further diagnostic or therapeutic measures to avoid disaster.

Coma and brain resuscitation

Coma is defined in the *Encyclopædia Britannica*[24] as:

> State of unconsciousness, characterized by loss of reaction to external stimuli and absence of spontaneous nervous activity, usually associated with injury to the cerebrum. Coma may accompany a number of metabolic disorders or physical injuries to the brain from disease or trauma.

The same source specifies **cardiopulmonary resuscitation (CPR)**[25] as an:

> Emergency procedure designed to restore normal breathing and circulation after such traumas as cardiac arrest and drowning. CPR involves clearing the air passages to the lungs and carrying out external heart massage by the exertion of pressure on the chest.

A person in a state of coma, regardless of its cause or duration, is in a life-threatening situation. As opposed to sleep, normal physiological defences such as the reflexes of coughing and swallowing may be absent when consciousness is lost. The likelihood of aspiration of saliva or vomitus creates perilous circumstances for a person whose brain may have already suffered oxygen deprivation or other detrimental effects. A person in coma is very dependent on others to protect his or her life. Coma is very common in conditions such as epilepsy, fainting, diabetes, stroke and head injury. Some of these conditions produce only temporary losses of consciousness (fainting, seizures) while others may result in a prolonged state of coma. The longer the coma the more complications can be anticipated, as is the case with stroke, head injury and drowning, for example.

There is a difference between basic, cardiopulmonary resuscitation (CPR) and brain resuscitation (CPCR).

> 1. Cardiopulmonary resuscitation or CPR is an emergency procedure, often employed after cardiac arrest, in which cardiac massage, artificial respiration, and drugs are used to maintain the circulation of oxygenated blood to the brain.

2. Cardiopulmonary-cerebral resuscitation CPCR is also an emergency measure which adds some additional considerations to CPR and continues as brain-oriented life support in the ICU. A healthy brain and a functional patient is the primary goal of cardiopulmonary-cerebral resuscitation. The essential reason for brain-oriented intensive care is the stabilization of **intracranial homeostasis**.

We will discuss in detail only CPCR, sometimes called Brain Resuscitation, which is a set of measures to prevent brain death and facilitate the survival of nerve cells.[26]

The concept of brain resuscitation is based on the premise that to secure ideal conditions for the brain, an operating condition called intracranial homeostasis is necessary to protect the nerve cells. A prerequisite to intracranial homeostasis is a normal supply of oxygen. Through respiration and the pumping action of the heart, life-sustaining oxygen must be carried to all organs including the brain.

In other words, a patient in coma either has to have natural heartbeat and breathing, or have restored heartbeat and breathing by cardiopulmonary resuscitation before brain resuscitation makes any sense. If, in the comatose person, the heartbeat and circulation are stabilized, the preconditions are present to begin brain-oriented life support or brain resuscitation.

Before going into brain resuscitation we should deal briefly with intracranial homeostasis.

Intracranial homeostasis, a steady state of functions, in simplified form can be characterized as follows.

The brain needs:

1. 3.3 ml of oxygen for each 100 gm of brain tissue every minute. The total need of the brain therefore is approximately 50 ml of oxygen per minute. If the oxygen supply is cut off through drowning or asphyxiation, the total oxygen content of the blood will be exhausted in approximately four to eight minutes.

2. a steady supply of blood sugar and a blood level of 80-120 mg of glucose for every 100 ml blood. The body's total glucose

reserve lasts for about two hours, following which hypoglycemia (low blood sugar) develops, resulting in serious derangement of brain functions leading to convulsions and coma.

3. a steady supply of blood. The **cerebral blood flow (CBF)**, has been established as 50 ml of blood for 100 gm of brain tissue every minute. Since the brain weighs about 1,500 gm (3 lb), the need for blood is about 750 ml (about 1.5 pints) per minute. This means that the total blood volume in the body recirculates through the brain once every seven minutes.

4. a continuous elimination of waste products of the body to maintain a normal hydrogen ion concentration (pH). The normal pH of the blood is slightly alkaline at 7.4. Deviation from this value can result in alkalosis or acidosis; both are harmful for brain functions and interfere with consciousness.

The brain also needs:

5. a normal pressure inside the skull to allow normal blood flow and good oxygen supply to the brain tissue. We have mentioned earlier, that a steady supply of oxygen through a steady **cerebral perfusion** and blood flow is needed by the brain cells for normal activity and survival. Cerebral perfusion depends on the difference between the **mean blood pressure** and brain tissue pressure (see **intracranial hypertension**). With a normal blood pressure of 120/80 mm Hg and a normal intracranial pressure of 10 mm Hg the **perfusion** pressure would be the ideal. If the blood pressure is low or the intracranial pressure is high, the perfusion pressure in the brain may be compromised. A cerebral perfusion pressure of less than 75 mm Hg is considered marginal for normal cell function. If the cerebral perfusion pressure sinks to 15 mm Hg, the blood and oxygen supply to the brain tissue becomes insufficient for nerve cell life.

From the above it should be obvious that maintenance of intracranial homeostasis is one of the most important demands on brain-oriented life support (CPCR) or brain resuscitation. If intracranial homeostasis cannot be maintained due to the seriousness of the insult to the brain or perhaps due to complications that may have developed during the first few hours of the illness or injury, the brain and particularly the nerve cells will undergo irreversible changes. This may not be compatible with recovery of consciousness and may preclude the indefinite maintenance of life support. We will expand on this later as we discuss the concept of irreversible coma, irreversible brain damage and brain death.

The diagnosis and management of coma

As there can be many causes of coma, so there are various degrees of depth in coma. Early diagnosis and effective treatment used at the right time may prevent death or irreversible damage to the brain (Guberman, 1982).[27]

In most cases the family physician will ask a specialist for a consultation. An internist or a neurologist and, in many instances, a neurosurgeon, will be asked to assist with the diagnosis and management of the comatose patient. Coma is always a medical or surgical emergency and it should be managed by a skilled team of health care personnel (Humphreys, 1982)[28] (Nelson, 1982).[29]

The first step in the management of coma is to make sure that the patient is breathing and that the heart is beating. This may involve cardiopulmonary resuscitation (CPR) followed by advanced cardiac or trauma life support and very often brain-oriented life support. Intravenous therapy will probably be started and monitoring equipment attached. Once the patient is stabilized, various blood tests and x-rays will be done. These may include radio-imaging of the brain with **computerized tomography (CT)**, **magnetic resonance imaging (MRI)** and/or positron emission tomography (**PET**) techniques.

The treatment will depend on the cause of coma. If conservative measures (drugs, hyperventilation) prove ineffective in normalizing a high intracranial pressure, surgery may be indicated to remove a blood clot or to perform a decompression craniotomy. To guide the optimal management of excessive pressure inside the skull, the placement of an intracranial pressure sensor may contribute to improving the mortality and morbidity of severe head injuries (Ivan et al., 1980).[30]

Fresh-water drowning is representative of that special circumstance when every effort should be made to resuscitate the victim, even though respiration and heartbeat may be absent and the individual may be "clinically dead". Several cases are known, both from the news and medical journals, of patients who, after 20-30 minutes of submersion, not only survived but walked out of the hospital a week or two later, apparently intact from every point of view. These survivals, almost without exception, have occurred in children who were rescued from cold or even icy water. In these cases, the water temperature may be the important factor in that it triggers the diving reflex (mammalian diving reflex) and thus saves the brain from damage.[31] The diving reflex mobilizes oxygenated blood from the peripheral parts of the body for use by the brain to support neuronal survival beyond the established limit of ten minutes.

After restarting the heart, these patients are usually treated with an artificially maintained low temperature (hypothermia) and drug-induced coma. These measures decrease the oxygen requirements of the nerve cells and may save billions of neurons struggling for survival. Since these patients are in deep coma with an abnormally low temperature even before treatment, hypothermia is considered one of the conditions when brain death criteria cannot be applied.

Since the early 1970s there has been an increasing effort to measure the depth of coma. Grading the depth of coma with a certain degree of accuracy helped to correlate the loss of consciousness with efficacy of treatment modalities as well as using the grades for their predictive values. One example of a frequently used grading method is the already discussed Glasgow Coma Scale (GCS), which gives a numerical denotation to the level of consciousness between three (the lowest, in deep, unresponsive coma) and fifteen (the highest, conscious, oriented and obeys commands well). Research has shown that if the score is three or four after twenty four hours, 87% of these patients will either die or remain in a **vegetative state**. In other words the coma score reflects the probability of recovery or the possible irreversibility and helps the physician to plan the treatment and the family to adjust to a hopeful or a guarded situation (Table III).

Table III

COMA AND SURVIVAL

G. C. S.	Responsiveness	Survival
3-5	Deep coma	Critical
6-8	Coma	Fair chance of survival
9-12	Stupor	Good chance of recovery
13-15	Drowsy	Excellent chance of recovery

The outcome from a comatose state depends on the nature of the insult to the brain and the length of time the nerve cells have been deprived of oxygen supply. The outcome is one of five distinct possibilities:

1. survival without any neurological or **cognitive** deficit,
2. survival with slight disability,
3. survival with moderate to severe disability,
4. survival in a vegetative state,
5. death.

Full recovery is often possible. If recovery is incomplete, the disability depends on the areas of the brain involved and the extent of the damage. If the whole cortex is damaged the highly controversial vegetative survival will occur. If both the cortex and the brainstem are destroyed, brain death is the result.

Survival without any deficit is the ideal outcome and it can, and does, happen in many cases, even in comatose states of long duration. We have seen many patients with severe head injuries who, though in coma for several days, recovered completely, without any serious neurological or psychological deficit. On the other hand, a prolonged coma of weeks or even months suggests that damage to the nerve cells was too extensive for the recovery and return of certain brain functions. (Bruce, 1982)[32] (Fischer, 2001)[33] (Demetriades, 2004)[34]

It is important to understand what is meant by irreversible damage as opposed to irreversible coma. Some patients recover from coma with motor deficits and/or mental or emotional changes caused by the irreversible damage to the nervous system. Others, following devastating and diffuse head injuries, are in an irreversible form of "**coma vigil**", or "chronic vegetative state" which precludes meaningful contact with the environment.

If the brain has been irrevocably damaged, life cannot be maintained despite total cardiac and respiratory support. It would seem that "life" and "death" coexist in an individual who is maintained by a mechanical ventilator and whose circulation is supported with drugs and oxygenation. Therefore, it becomes a matter of definition and established criteria whether or not a person on total artificial "life support" is indeed alive or dead. When the coma is irreversible, the patient's heart would stop if the body and the heart were not oxygenated by the use of the mechanical respirator.

The use of strict criteria in these cases establishes with great accuracy that the brain and brainstem have been damaged to such an extent that survival of the person is not possible. The diagnosis of brain death is final; it means that life has ended without any chance of revival. It is an irreversible condition that is diagnosed by universally approved criteria. After the diagnosis of brain death, (unless transplantation is being considered) respiratory support becomes pointless. The resuscitation restarted the heart, but failed to restart the brain because the nerve cells that maintain consciousness and breathing are more sensitive to oxygen deprivation than the cells in the heart.

In spite of its use for over fifty years, the term "brain death" still remains controversial. With other related issues, e.g. transplantation protocols, vegetative survival and **euthanasia**, the debate is evident among ethicist, legal and religious authorities as well as in various publications in medical literature, the media and the courts. Interestingly, those who have never seen a dead patient on the respirator or patients in a vegetative state seem to be the main source

of critical doubts about brain death and its concept and definition
from a legal, religious or ethical point of view. Conversely, those who
work with these unfortunate patients routinely seem to find these
new criteria useful, perhaps because they seem to answer practical
needs at the bedside without trivializing the solemnity of dying and
the painful reality of death.

Notes

1. Veatch, R. M., *Death, Dying and the Biological Revolution: Our last quest for
responsibility* (New Haven: Yale University Press, 1977).
This is an excellent, rational discussion of many aspects of death.

2. Hoffman, J., *The Life and Death of Cells* (New York: Doubleday and Company,
1957).
A biophysicist and cancer researcher explains how cells grow, divide, organize in
tissue and die.

3. Safar, P., (ed.), Brain resuscitation, *Crit Care Med, Special Issue*, 6, (1978):
199-291.
Highly technical text, suitable only for readers with medical background.

4. Ventureyra, E., Ivan, L. P., Brain resuscitation (special communication), *Can J
Neurol Sci*, 6, (1979): 71-72.

5. Harvey, W., *Exercitatio anatomica de motu cordis et sanguinis in animalibus*
(An Anatomical Exercise on the Motion of the Heart and Blood in Animals),
(1628).

6. Royal Humane Society <http://www.scholarly-societies.org/history/1774rhs.
html>, accessed August 20, 2006.
The Society was founded by two doctors who wanted to promote the new, but
controversial, medical technique of resuscitation.

7. Black, H., *Black's Law Dictionary*, 4th edn. (St. Paul, MN: West Publishing
Co.,1951).

8. *Dorland's Illustrated Medical Dictionary*, 23rd edn. (Philadelphia: W. B.
Saunders, 1957).

9. Safar, P., On the history of modern resuscitation, *Crit Care Med*, 24, (2 Suppl.),
(1996): S3-S11.

10. Pope Pius XII, The Prolongation of Life: Allocution to the International Congress of Anesthesiologists, November 24, 1957, in *The Pope Speaks*, Vol. 4, (1958): 393-398.

11. Mollaret, P., Goulon, M., Le coma dépassé, *Rev Neurol*, 101, (1959): 5-15.

12. Report of the Ad Hoc Committee of the Harvard Medical School to examine the definition of brain death. A definition of irreversible coma, *JAMA*, 205(6) (1968): 337-340.

13. Adrian, E., Bremer, F., Jasper, H. H., (eds.), *Brain Mechanism and Consciousness* (Oxford: Blackwell, 1964).

14. Adam, G., *Perception, Consciousness, Memory: Reflections of a biologist* (New York: Plenum Press, 1980).

15. Davidson, J. M., Davidson, R. J., (eds.), *The Psychobiology of Consciousness* (New York: Plenum Press, 1980).

16. Furst, C., Consciousness and brain processes, in id., *Origins of the Mind* (Englewood Cliffs, NJ: Prentice-Hall, 1979): 197-216.

17. Searle, J., *The Mystery of Consciousness* (New York: New York Review of Books, Inc., 1997).

18. Flanagan, O., *The Science of the Mind* (Cambridge, MA: MIT Press, 1993).

19. McKinney, L. O., *Neurotheology: Virtual religion in the 21ˢᵗ century* (Cambridge, MA: American Institute for Mindfulness, 1994).

20. Magoun, H. W., An ascending reticular activating system in the brainstem, *Arch Neurol Psychiat*, 67, (1952): 145-154.

21. Teasdale, G., Jennett, B., Assessment of coma and impaired consciousness: A practical scale, *Lancet*, 2, (1974): 81-84.

22. Lombardi, F., Taricco, M., De Tanti, A., et al., Sensory stimulation of brain-injured individuals in coma or vegetative state: Results of a Cochrane systematic review, *Clin Rehabil*, 16(5), (2002): 464-472.

23. Berger, E., Vavrick, K., Hochgatterer, P., Vigilance scoring in children with acquired brain injury: Vienna Vigilance Score in comparison with usual coma scales, *J Child Neurol*, 16(4), (2001): 236-240.

24. coma in *Encyclopædia Britannica* <http://www.britannica.com/eb/article-9024905>, accessed April 15, 2006.

25. cardiopulmonary resuscitation in *Encyclopædia Britannica* <http://www.britannica.com/eb/article-9020301>, accessed May 16, 2006.

26. Safar, P., Bircher, N. G., *Cardiopulmonary-Cerebral Resuscitation: An introduction to resuscitation medicine*. World Federation of Societies of Anesthesiologists, 3rd edn., (Stavanger: Laerdal, 1988).
The book is easy to understand and suitable for readers without medical background.

27. Guberman, A., Coma as a neurological emergency, in L. P. Ivan, D. A. Bruce, (eds.), *Coma: Physiopathology, diagnosis and management* (Springfield, IL: Charles C. Thomas, 1982): 283-317.

28. Humphreys, P., Coma in infancy and childhood, in L. P. Ivan, D. A. Bruce, (eds.), *Coma: Physiopathology, diagnosis and management* (Springfield, IL: Charles C. Thomas, 1982): 102-125.

29. Nelson, R., Coma in cereberovascular disease in L. P. Ivan, D. A. Bruce, (eds.), *Coma: Physiopathology, diagnosis and management* (Springfield, IL: Charles C. Thomas, 1982): 126-139.

30. Ivan, L. P., Ventureyra, E. C. G., Choo, S., Intracranial pressure monitoring with the fiber optic transducer in children, *Child's Brain*, 7, (1980): 303-313.
The evidence suggested that monitoring intracranial pressure reduces the mortality and morbidity of traumatic brain injury.

31. "A reflexive response to diving in many aquatic mammals and birds, characterized by physiological changes that decrease oxygen consumption, such as slowed heart rate and decreased blood flow to the abdominal organs and muscles, until breathing resumes. Though less pronounced, the reflex also occurs in certain nonaquatic animals, including humans, upon submersion in water." *American Heritage Dictionaries* <http://www.answers.com/topic/mammalian-diving-reflex>, accessed April 26, 2006.

32. Bruce, D. A., Coma grading systems and the outcome of coma in L. P. Ivan, D. A. Bruce, (eds.), *Coma: Physiopathology, diagnosis and management* (Springfield, IL: Charles C. Thomas, 1982): 140-146.

33. Fischer, J., Mathieson, C., The history of the Glasgow Coma Scale: Implications for practice, *Crit Care Nurs Q*, 23(4), (2001):52-58.

34. Demetriades, D., Kuncir, E., et al., Outcome and prognostic factors in head injuries with an admission Glasgow Coma Scale score of 3, *Arch Surg* 139(10), (2004): 1066-1068.

CHAPTER 2
BRAIN DEATH

There are several ways to define "brain death". A paper in the Canadian Medical Association Journal (Lazar et al., 2001) defines brain death as the "complete and irreversible absence of all brain function".[1]

The *Concise Oxford English Dictionary* formulates it this way:

> brain death, n. irreversible brain damage causing the end of independent respiration.

Since the control centres for essential functions such as consciousness and respiration are located within the brainstem there is a trend, particularly in the UK, to replace the term "brain death" with **"brainstem death"**.[2]

Kuchta recently dealt with the problem of brain death vs. brainstem death (Kuchta, 2004)[3] and pointed out that although modern technology has produced an entity widely known as brain death, a conceptual and terminological crisis still exists.

Evolution of the concept

The concept of brain death evolved when the traditional criteria of death could not solve the terrible dilemma of failed resuscitation.

To understand the situation more fully, try to imagine the following scenario: The year is 1964; a close relative has suffered a heart attack. The heart is restarted successfully after ten minutes of cardiac arrest. In the course of resuscitation our relative is **intubated** and put on the respirator which oxygenates the body and the heart.

The heart, now beating spontaneously, carries oxygen to all organs. Seemingly every organ performs its normal duty; the liver and the kidneys get rid of waste products from the blood and eliminate bile and urine; the skin sweats; the bowels move and the whole digestive system absorbs nourishment from the food provided by tubes into the stomach.

This would appear to have been a successful resuscitation procedure. The heart is beating and circulation of the blood is restored but, unfortunately, the life-saving efforts came a few minutes late and the brain could not tolerate this length of oxygen starvation. Since all the nerve cells suffered extreme and irreversible damage, the brain as an organ, has become a severely damaged tissue, with necrosis in areas that are necessary for consciousness and respiration.

If the brain is dead and a patient is kept on the respirator for twenty-four hours or more (to satisfy medical regulations for example), a gamut of abnormalities can be seen at autopsy. These abnormalities range from focal infarctions or hemorrhages, to complete disintegration and partial liquefaction of the contents of the skull. The brain is sometimes so friable that it falls apart when attempts are made to remove it at post-mortem examination. In extreme cases the cranial cavity can be filled with semiliquid **autolysed detritus**. Microscopic examination reveals widespread disintegration of the neurons and those that remain exhibit very severe changes, incompatible with any degree of function.

This patient may have looked like other patients in a lighter coma, except for the fact that neurological examination showed no measurable brain function. This allowed for the conclusion that a) because of the irreversible destruction of the **respiratory centre** the patient will never be able to breathe spontaneously and b) there will be no interaction with the environment, not even a blink of the eye, no swallowing of saliva or food and no cough reflex because the cerebral cortex and the brainstem were also destroyed. The lost neurons contained not only the memory of the system but also the programme which makes the system work. Our relative, in the absence of functioning nerve cells in the brain, cannot think and cannot feel even though the pain-carrying nerve fibres may be intact in the spinal cord, below the brainstem. Using extraordinary measures, this condition may prevail for several weeks or months until the whole system slowly falters and a final cardiac arrest terminates the artificially maintained "life".

In the late Fifties and early Sixties a number of patients, like our relative in the above scenario, started to appear in hospitals. (Note that we are not talking about the "vegetative state" in which the patient is able to breathe.) Here we are describing an irreversible coma without spontaneous breathing when a mechanical respirator pumps air into the lungs, and the heart in turn oxygenates the organs of the body. Doctors, faced with this situation, did not know what their moral obligation was or how long they were supposed to continue artificial maintenance. The patient's condition was not only hopeless but, as experience would show, totally irreversible.

Anxious relatives around the bedside were equally disturbed. At first they wanted everything possible done to save the life of a loved one but, as time went on, the vigil became more and more painful. The prolonged maintenance of patients in deep coma meant more tubes and wires and increasing difficulties with the life support system. The kidneys began to fail, the blood pressure and the body temperature slowly dropped. For a while, corrections were possible, but our imaginary relative would be bruised, cold, and **cyanotic** and look more and more like a **cadaver**. All the while the respirator would continue pumping and the heart continue to beat. However, blood was not circulating into the brain because the swollen disintegrating brain tissue had created pressure gradients higher than the force of the circulating blood. The scene was devastating for the relatives who had to accept hopelessness, and extremely difficult for the nursing staff in continuing the futile care of a lifeless body.

Doctors in the late Fifties and the early Sixties did not have a clear answer, although most of them knew that to keep an essentially dead person on the respirator was morally wrong. The futile effort was not only expensive in terms of equipment and nursing care, but prolonged the suffering of despondent relatives and deprived other patients, who could have been helped with the use of a respirator, because in those years the number of respirators was usually limited even in the most sophisticated hospitals.

French anesthesiologists and neurologists took it upon themselves to refer this dilemma to the Pope, who was considered by them to be the highest moral and religious authority, to resolve this problem to the satisfaction of doctors, patients and relatives. By this time, accumulated autopsy evidence revealed extensive necrotic changes in the brain of patients who died after failed resuscitation. This pathology, first thought to be the result of respirator use, was called "respirator brain".[4] Through research and consultation pathologists soon recognized that the death of the brain must have been the cause of unresponsive coma and the extended use of the respirator was the consequence of a lifeless brain.

It was in 1957 that Pope Pius XII answered the French physicians' questions about moral and religious obligations in irreversible coma (Pope Pius XII, 1958).[5] He said that the obligation, according to Christian morality, is to use ordinary means (as opposed to extraordinary means, that is, life support), ". . . since these forms of treatment go beyond the ordinary means to which one is bound, it cannot be held that there is an obligation to use them". In discussing irreversible coma, the Pope stated: "It remains for the doctor . . . to give a clear and precise definition of death and the 'moment of death' of a patient who passes away in a state of unconsciousness. Here one can accept the usual concept of complete and final separation of the soul from the body". (page 396, paragraph 3)

Before the time of modern resuscitation, cardiac and respiratory arrest (now reversible syndromes) were chosen as the signs of cessation of vital functions. Since the absence of respiration was frequently observed as the final event of dying, it was justifiable to talk about the moment of death. Similarly, the disappearance of heartbeat or the absence of pulse was relatively easy to monitor and use as another sign of death. Physicians and even lay coroners were easily trained to observe the absence of respiration, heartbeat and other "infallible" signs (rigor mortis, coldness of the body, lividity on the dependent parts and so on), which established that death had occurred.

With the newer techniques of life support, some of these signs become meaningless. For example, the heartbeat can be re-established by CPR in acute situations and the use of a mechanical respirator may go on for weeks and months without the return of spontaneous breathing and consciousness. For these reasons a new concept of death had to evolve; a concept which would be approved by the law and accepted by scientists, doctors and philosophers.

An acceptable definition

The main problem in the late Fifties and early Sixties was to define brain death as a syndrome; that is, to group characteristic signs and set up standard requirements for the diagnosis of irreversible coma. This type of coma would ultimately become the new brain-oriented definition of death.

Another vexing problem was that determination of the moment of death, among these new conditions, became a rather ill-defined time. Rather than seeing death as an easily definable moment or a sharp change that would clearly indicate how and when life ended, doctors learned that death was a gradual process.

With the newer concept of death and the gradual acceptance of brain death as the death of a person, the diagnosis of the absence of life functions became more complicated than ever. The complexity of the diagnostic work required the expertise of two neurologically-oriented specialists (neurologists or neurosurgeons) who were not only familiar with brain function but also with the equipment used to establish the diagnosis of irreversible coma. The decision of whether, in all certainty, the coma was irreversible took time because two specialists had to agree that brain death had indeed occurred.

The clinical criteria of brain death emerged from the original attempts to define irreversible coma. The historical statements of the World Medical Assembly in Sydney, August 9, 1968 (Appendix A) and in the same year the **Harvard criteria** of irreversible coma[6] indelibly influenced medical ethics, biological thinking and the law.

There have been modifications to the original Harvard criteria but the validity of irreversible coma as an acceptable definition of death has been respected by medical, religious and ethical thinkers like Skegg (1984),[7] Veatch (1989)[8] and Tooley (1979).[9]

The universally accepted criteria of brain death are:

1. Unresponsive coma
2. Inability to breathe spontaneously
3. Absence of **brainstem reflexes**
4. Absence of electrical activity of the brain (the so-called **isoelectric EEG**), which is not obligatory among certain conditions

An excellent definition of brain death was issued by the honorary secretary of the Conference of Medical Royal Colleges and their Faculties in the United Kingdom in 1976 and 1979 (see Appendix B for further study).

Medical limitations

These new developments in medicine were at first controversial. A understanding of the issues needed validation by establishing that the new concept of death based on brain-oriented criteria was more accurate than the traditional definitions of death.

Firstly, it was not difficult to prove that the diagnosis of death by old methods, as had been ascertained by inspection of the body, feeling the pulse and listening to the heart, can be inaccurate. Numerous cases were reported for many years about persons pronounced dead on the street or at home by a qualified physician and later found snoring in one of the city morgues.

Apart from the inaccuracy of the traditional method of declaring somebody dead, these criteria had become obsolete for another reason. The cessation of heartbeat was no longer a sign of death; rather it became a medical emergency called cardiac arrest. Similarly, the cessation of respiration ceased to be the evidence of lifelessness and became another emergency known as respiratory arrest.

If heartbeat can be restarted and respiration can be maintained by a respirator what then is the reason for unsuccessful cardiopulmonary resuscitation? What is the difference between those who survive resuscitation and those who do not? What kind of damage to which organ makes revival of a person impossible? Though much can be done to help an individual survive an episode when the brain has been compromised, as happens many times following drowning, stroke and cardiac arrest, survival depends on the time and extent of brain damage. If the damage is limited and the elapsed time is compatible with survival of the neurons, resuscitation is successful. If the cells of the brain are irreversibly damaged, the brain cannot be restarted and efforts of revival would certainly fail.

The success of kidney and heart replacement triggered wishful thinking about brain transplantation with the suggestion that if the destroyed brain could be restarted or replaced, the question of immortality would be solved. But, as we will show, the brain cannot be replaced and the reason for this is not only technical but primarily philosophical, and it concerns the identity of a person.

To understand the above statement try to imagine an advanced transplantation system that allows every component of the body to be replaced with either new mechanical or used human parts. This advance in science would mean that one by one every organ in the body could be renewed. Arteriosclerotic arteries could be mended, cirrhotic livers and diseased kidneys replaced, and ultimately every diseased, aged or malfunctioning organ could be exchanged for a machine, a new organ from a fresh human cadaver or from the body of an animal.

The only stubborn obstacle to total transplantation of body parts in the above illustration is the brain. It does not lend itself easily to transplantation because of the extreme complexity of anatomy and the intricacy of blood supply, not to mention the unsolved problem of cranial nerve regeneration, without which a new brain would not be able to operate the body.

Granted, it is possible to imagine that one day all twelve **cranial nerves** on each side of the brainstem could be sutured and made to regenerate; all vessels could be sutured and kept patent; the spinal cord could be sewn to the brainstem and the millions of fibres made to regenerate and grow into the spinal cord to find and revitalize specific nerve cells and muscle fibres in the body. Only then would transplantation of the brain or the head, if you wish, be a real possibility.

But who would be the donor? A healthy young man? Let us suppose that such a brain would be available and the transplantation would take place with all the necessary regeneration of the millions of nerve fibres. What would be the identity of the "new" individual? In this case the individual who survives would be the donor, bringing his memory, life experience and personality into an old and diseased body. The personality of the recipient would disappear. The young man who "donated" his brain would have "gained" an old dilapidated body which will not be able to serve his needs. Such a donation is impossible to imagine. Similarly, the brain of a non-human primate would be of little help to a demented old gentleman because, as the recipient, he would disappear and the monkey would survive in a rickety old human body.

We have to recognize and accept the notion that the brain cannot be transplanted because the person is inseparable from it. The human being is his brain. Thoughts, feelings, idiosyncrasies, miseries and personality—all are in the brain. The "I" is not transferable. The irreplaceable brain is the final obstacle to physical immortality. The death of the brain, therefore, will always remain the irreversible aspect of a person's death.

Controversies about the time of death

The relationship between body and soul, one of the ultimate questions, clearly divides philosophies. Idealism and materialism, as well as the great religions of the world, have differing views on the subject. The interpretation of death, concerning both physical existence and the understanding of what survives the individual after the termination of life, is also a great divider.

Theists would say that the soul leaves the body at the moment of death and may go to heaven, hell or purgatory, depending on religious affiliation and belief. Materialists would say that only offspring, creations in art and science, and memories which live in others, survive physical death.

Whatever our belief might be, the brain appears to be the organ which processes information in all animals, including man. Therefore, it would seem to be the instrument of the soul. It is the tool which forms and expresses love, hatred, good and bad intentions, spirituality and the lack of it; the brain is the guidance system of our whole response to life and to the environment, our physical, intellectual and spiritual existence. When the brain dies, experience must cease and, as Pope Pius XII stated, in deep coma, the soul may have already left the body. It is, therefore, appropriate, both from the spiritual and physiological point of view, to designate the moment of brain death as the most characteristic marker of the time of death.

From the foregoing thoughts it might appear that the determination of the time of death has now been simplified. When the patient passes over the threshold from life to death, particularly in a sophisticated tertiary care unit where equipment and expertise are available for making accurate and foolproof diagnostic statements, determination of the time of death must be adroit and accurate.[10] Unfortunately this is not the case, because of the new insight that death is a gradual process. Physicians can affirm with confidence and with scientifically accumulated proof that brain death has occurred. However, to reach this certainty a number of tests must be performed over a specified time period before it is possible to state that a coma which at 10 a.m. appeared reversible and treatable, a few hours later has turned into an irreversible devastation of the brain which cannot be improved in spite of the fact that some **spinal reflexes** may be present.[11]

> **Case history.** A 42-year-old nurse was brought to the hospital in deep coma. She was breathing spontaneously but had fixed dilated pupils. After energetic brain resuscitation, the pupils began to react to light and after **endotracheal intubation** she was taken to the radiology department for a CT scan. The CT scan disclosed a brain hemorrhage not amenable to surgical treatment.

The findings were explained to her husband who understood that the situation was grave but not entirely hopeless; recovery remained a remote possibility. For the best management of increased intracranial pressure a sensor was implanted under the skull to monitor the pressure continuously. The very high intracranial pressure (ICP) of 70 mm Hg responded to treatment reasonably well and within two hours the intracranial pressure was reduced to 40 mm Hg and the condition of the patient was more stable. One hour later a sudden drop of blood pressure occurred without detectable reason and could not be corrected in time. Because the blood pressure and intracranial pressure readings were of similar value, the brain was not being perfused with blood for a sufficiently long time to suspect that brain death might have occurred.

An electroencephalogram (EEG) was performed and the tracing was "flat" or without brainwaves. This lack of electrical activity in the brain is known as **electrocerebral silence** and is one of the characteristic signs of brain death.

The findings were disclosed to her husband. He fully understood that further treatment was pointless and that now, the diagnosis of brain death was to be established through consultation and further confirmatory tests. The husband, devastated by the news, wished to terminate artificial maintenance as soon as possible. A second opinion was requested and this consultant immediately ordered another EEG because he was not satisfied with the quality of the record. The consultant concurred with the diagnosis of brain death but to satisfy protocol, it was necessary to repeat the EEG twelve hours after the first one. Therefore, it was not until the next day that agreement was reached that brain death had occurred. It had taken less than two hours on the day of admission to establish that a treatable condition had become an irreversible coma and more than twenty-four hours to establish brain death.

Because of the complexity of the problem, which involves not only the use of sophisticated equipment but the efforts of two consultants, the so-called moment of death becomes a matter of diagnostic agreement between two experts. In fact, this may occur several hours after the "moment" of biological death, or the death of the brain.

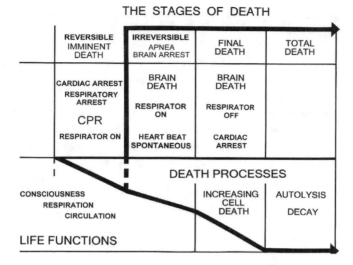

Fig. 3. *The diagram illustrates the overlap between life and death. With the increasing process of cell death, life functions gradually decrease during the various stages of death.*

The so-called time of death has always been an arbitrary moment within an overlapping segment of decreasing vital functions and increasing quantity of cell death (Fig. 3). Since the invention of mechanical respirators, we have learned to see this overlap in slow motion and to recognize, with other biological scientists, that death is a gradual process. No matter how convenient it is to assume that death and life are opposite and that a patient is either dead or alive, the process of death is a gradual event and organs die at different rates depending on their resistance to the lack of oxygen.

The dying process of the brain itself is gradual. Depending on the resistance of various cell structures and on the length of time during which oxygen supply to the brain was lacking, the function of the cortex and the brainstem may be extinguished at a different rate. As a result, death cannot be a moment, as the law believes; it is and always has been an arbitrary line within an overlapping segment of decreasing cell functions and increasing cell death.

The law and the criteria of death

The law does not originate new concepts but, if a new concept is accepted by society as ethical, the law makers seek integration of ethical concepts into social codes.

The old criteria, as dictated by the earlier concept of death, were all based on the absence of respiratory and cardiac function. Changes to the law have taken several years and there are still countries, states or provinces that have no legal definition of brain death. Various countries have dealt with the problem quite differently, as seen in the following brief comparative summary.

In the United States of America, the state of Kansas enacted a statute in 1971 which served as a model for other American states. The statute recognizes brain death but does not impose medical tests for its determination.

In Canada, the first province to enact a brain-oriented definition of death was Manitoba, in 1974, stating that "for all purposes within the legislative competence of the Legislature of Manitoba, the death of a person takes place at a time at which irreversible cessation of all that person's brain function occurs".

In Great Britain, lawyers and doctors generally opposed legislative intervention, although the Conference of Medical Colleges recognized and approved the concept of brain death and suggested clearly defined criteria in determining death with brain-oriented tests (Appendix B).

In preparation for a federal law, the Law Reform Commission of Canada submitted a report to Parliament in 1981. The Commission recommended the following definition of death:

1. A person is dead when an irreversible cessation of all that person's brain functions has occurred.
2. The irreversible cessation of brain functions can be determined by the prolonged absence of spontaneous circulatory and respiratory functions.
3. When the determination of the prolonged absence of spontaneous circulatory and respiratory functions is made impossible by the use of artificial means of support, the

irreversible cessation of brain functions can be determined by any means recognized by the ordinary standards of current medical practice.[12]

As of 2007, this recommendation had not been enacted into federal law.

The wording of the U.S. Federal Task Force is similar:

Uniform Determination of Death Act. "An individual who has sustained either (1) irreversible cessation of circulatory and respiratory functions or (2) irreversible cessation of all functions of the entire brain including the brainstem, is dead. A determination of death must be made in accordance with accepted medical standards." (See Appendix D for details.)

Irreversible coma and brain death

These two concepts are not identical from a medical or legal point of view. Irreversible coma is a medical diagnosis which can be tentatively made, based on certain clinical criteria, whereas brain death is backed by law, provided a pronouncement is based on the specific requirements of current medical standards in a country.

The following short discussion and the case studies should illustrate the point and assist with the understanding of the difference between these two terms.

Irreversible coma simply means that such extensive damage has occurred to the brain, usually after brain hemorrhage or head injury, that recovery to a conscious state is not possible.[13] Some of these patients may die without respiratory support; others may live for months or years in a vegetative state.

Brain death, on the other hand, means that maintenance of tissue oxygenation without respiratory support is not possible. Even with prolonged use of the mechanical respirator, consciousness cannot return and heart activity cannot be maintained indefinitely.[14]

Both conditions result from extensive damage to the brain but, in brain death both the cognitive and the vital centres (the cortex and the brainstem) are destroyed.

In brain death there is no spontaneous respiration upon discontinuation of mechanical ventilation, whereas, in irreversible coma with vegetative survival, breathing will continue.

Both in brain death and in irreversible coma (coma vigil or **persistent vegetative state**) the patients have no future hope of communicating with the environment. However in vegetative survival, sleep (eyes closed without normal sleep patterns on the EEG) will alternate with wakefulness (eyes open, swallowing and cough reflexes present, but no interaction with the environment can be observed or elicited), hence the term "coma vigil".

Case history 1. This case is similar to the now famous Karen Ann Quinlan story. A 24-year-old single woman is on the respirator following severe encephalitis which has affected the whole brain except for the brainstem. The EEG is flat and clinically she exists only at a brainstem level. She is able to breathe a little but needs assisted ventilation. Six weeks after the onset of her illness, she shows no evidence of progress. The doctor informs the family that according to the CT scan findings, the EEG and other tests, she has evidence of irreversible brain damage and will never recover from coma. After an extensive consultation, members of the family decide that prolongation of life among these conditions is unfair and they wish to terminate the use of the respirator.

The attending neurologist assures the family that he is in full sympathy with them, and if the person were his sister he would wish for her to be taken off the respirator, but he cannot do this. According to present medical standards, the patient is alive and her treatment requires respiratory support.

The family consults a lawyer and on his advice they go to court. A court injunction instructs the doctor to terminate treatment. The attending physician "pulls the plug". The patient starts breathing on her own, first with great inefficiency but gradually more regularly and efficiently. She continues her existence in coma in a so-called chronic vegetative state. She will live as long as good nursing and medical care is able to prevent complications that commonly occur in coma.

In this case there was irreversible brain damage but, in the absence of the strict criteria of brain death, the doctor, as a matter of conscience and professional integrity, refused to discontinue supportive care. Indeed, in spite of the court order, the patient did not die. Her coma was irreversible but because of the incomplete destruction of the brain she was able to breathe on her own.

Case history 2. A 16-year-old boy, hit by a car while riding his bicycle, is in deep coma four hours after the injury. The CT scan shows several bruises and hemorrhages in the brain, the EEG is flat, and an ICP monitoring device reads a brain pressure of 110 while the **systolic** blood pressure is only 70 mm Hg. The patient is on a respirator, the body temperature is falling, and the pupils are fixed and dilated.

There is a consultation between the family and the attending neurosurgeon. He informs them that the situation is grave because the boy has suffered irreversible brain damage and, in fact, he believes that the brain is dead. Therefore, the next day, after a confirmation of the findings, a consultation and a second EEG, he might suggest discontinuation of life support.

The mother is desperate and would like to do something more radical, suggesting that, even if the chance of survival is one in a million, she would like to have surgery done to relieve the pressure on the brain. There is a long compassionate discussion and the doctor explains that everything possible was done; all supportive treatment will continue and there is no chance of helping the boy to survive if the brain and the brainstem are irreversibly destroyed. The family asks for a second opinion. Another neurosurgeon reviews the findings, sees the patient and agrees that brain death has occurred and surgery would only cause further suffering for the family without changing a hopeless situation.

The family now decides that they would like to have life support stopped immediately if the boy is dead. To his regret, the neurosurgeon has to say that hospital regulations and protocol demand that a second EEG must be done twelve hours after the first. Therefore, he has to continue life support for several hours and only after the second EEG can the patient be taken off the respirator. The family accepts this and as their son's life cannot be saved they consent to donation of the kidneys or whatever organ may be needed to help somebody else. The boy himself, a few months earlier, had expressed his support of organ transplantation.

The next day the EEG is repeated, an **apnea test** is performed; the young man is examined neurologically and all criteria of brain death are present. He is pronounced dead and transferred to the operating room. After the pronouncement of death he is under the custody of the transplant team who are totally independent from the treating physicians. The transplant team complete the removal of the kidneys and the corneas and turns off the respirator. The heartbeat is monitored and after about twenty minutes the heart stops and the time is recorded as the time of cardiac arrest.

In this case, the boy was in irreversible coma with brain death and this removes the professional, ethical and legal obligation to continue treatment.

In October 1985, Pope John Paul II received in audience a group of scientists assembled at the invitation of the Pontifical Academy of Sciences to discuss the themes: "The Artificial Prolongation of Life and the Determination of the Exact Moment of Death." The result of this consensus was reported in a monograph (Chagas, 1986).[15] This 114-page booklet contains valuable information from Carlos Chagas, President of the Pontifical Academy of Sciences, Vatican City, and other leading neuroscientists of the decade from the United States, West Germany, Brazil, Sweden, France, Italy and the Netherlands.

Pope John Paul II, addressing this distinguished working group, made—among other comments—the following statement:

When inevitable death is imminent in spite of the means used, it is permitted in conscience to take the decision to refuse forms of treatment that would only secure a precarious and burdensome prolongation of life . . .

After a three-day meeting in October 1985, the conclusions summarized the issues as follows:

> *Definition of death:* A person is dead when he has suffered irreversible loss of all capacity for integrating and coordinating physical and mental functions of the body.
> Death has occurred when:
> a) Spontaneous cardiac and respiratory functions have irreversibly ceased, or
> b) There has been an irreversible cessation of all brain functions.
>
> *Medical guidelines:* If the patient is in permanent coma, irreversible as far as it is possible to predict, treatment is not required, but care, including feeding, must be provided.
> If some prospect of recovery is medically established, treatment is also required or pursued.
> If treatment may bring no benefit to the patient, it can be withdrawn, care being pursued.
> By "care" the Working Group considers the ordinary help due to bedridden patients, as well as compassion and affective and spiritual support due to every human being in danger.

Brain death worldwide

We have already discussed the legal status of brain death in Canada, the UK and in the USA and found striking similarities in the legal definitions and the medical criteria of death in the three countries. In an editorial in *Neurology* the author points out (Swash, 2002)[16] that "There is uneasy conflict between the rationalist view that death occurs when the brain is dead, and the differing view— which must command respect–that death of the whole organism is the final moment in a person's life".

In our search for information we have found that the legal status of brain death is not yet complete in the world. Nevertheless, one outstanding paper (Wijdicks, 2002)[17] gives a fair estimate.

Wijdicks has found that legal standards on brain death and organ transplantation were present in 55 of 80 surveyed countries (69%). Practice guidelines for adults were in effect in 70 of 80 countries (88%), only about half of which recommended apnea testing. Confirmatory laboratory testing was mandatory in 28% of practice guidelines.

There is an astounding variation in the dates when brain death and transplantation were regulated or approved by some of the countries. In China, for example (China Internet Information Centre, 2004),[18] the Ministry of Health approved the first standard in 2004 on how to determine brain death accurately. The standard was formulated in 2003 by the Tongji Hospital.

In Denmark, opinion polls have heightened public unease with physician-declared brain death. In one paper, Jorgensen (1996)[19] pointed out that criteria of brain death had been disputed in Denmark for more than twenty years before the Danish Parliament in 1990 finally passed a law on declaration of death, postmortem examination and transplantation of organs. The new law introduced criteria of brain death as supplementary to the criteria of cardiac death. Denmark became one of the last of the European countries to legalize criteria of brain death.

Information was sporadic until Wijdicks' paper triggered a flurry of correspondence from around the world. Brain death regulation was passed by Taiwan in 1987, the former Yugoslavia in 1980 and most recently Serbia in 1996. In Italy an earlier law from 1975 has been replaced by a new law, which was formulated in 1993 and accepted in 1999.

In France, the laws—enforced respectively in 1968, 1978, 1991 and 1996—provided a framework for brain-death criteria for organ transplantation and included EEG recording. Huet confirmed in 1996 that the legal definition of brain death in France is based on electroencephalographic criteria in patients with clinical evidence of irreversible coma. (Huet et al., 1996)[20] However, since certain conditions (the use of sedative drugs, low body temperature) may render the EEG unreliable, it becomes necessary to prove the lack of blood flow to the brain. This can be achieved by certain time-comsuming methods (e.g. **angiography**, CT scan, etc.). Huet and his co-authors prefer a digitized intra-arterial cerebral **parenchymography**. This simple fast technique does not alter physiological conditions and provides high-quality images, ensuring prompt diagnosis, which is a prerequisite for optimal organ removal.

Among Islamic countries, six out of nine have a legal definition of brain death. The latest statement by the Council of Islamic Jurisprudence, which includes jurists from all schools of thought in Islam and which meets regularly to review some of these new rulings, reads as follows:

> It is permissible to switch off the life support system with total and irreversible loss of function of the whole brain in a patient if three attending specialist physicians render their opinion unequivocally that irreversible cessation of brain functions has occurred. This is so even when the essential functions of the heart and the lungs are externally supported by life support system. However, legal death cannot be pronounced except when the vital functions have ceased after the external support system has been switched off (Sachedina, 2005).[21]

Germany has adopted brain death for the diagnosis of death. The following criteria are listed in a paper by Thomke and Weilemann, (2000).[22]

> . . . The intervals of a repeat clinical evaluation are at least 12 hours in patients with primary, and at least 72 hours in those with secondary, brain damage.
> Electroencephalography documented absence of electrical activity for at least 30 minutes or by means of intracranial Doppler **ultrasonography** or **isotope angiography** documented intracranial circulatory arrest also confirm brain death.

Confirmatory tests are not mandatory in most cases but required in newborns, infants below the age of two years, and patients with **infratentorial** brain damage.

Japan adopted brain death criteria in 1997, (Masahiro Morioka, 2001).[23] The law allows people to choose between traditional death and brain death. Organ transplantation from brain-dead bodies can occur only if acceptance of brain death was recorded on his or her donor card.

As we have shown and confirmed by others earlier (Haupt and Rudolf, 1999),[24] the majority of European countries have published recommendations for the diagnosis of brain death as a necessary prerequisite for organ donation. The concept of brain death and its definition are generally accepted in all of Europe; however, the guidelines for determining the total and irreversible loss of all brain functions differ somewhat among the various countries. While the clinical examination and documentation of the clinical signs of brain death are very similar, there are significant differences in the guidelines for using technical confirmatory tests to corroborate the clinical signs. These range from rejecting all technical tests to the acceptance of multiple neurophysiological tests alone or in combination. The diagnosis of brain death is based on a number of prerequisites, namely:

- the clinical diagnosis of deep coma,
- loss of all brainstem reflexes, and
- the demonstration of apnea.

Neurophysiological tests are recommended by a number of national professional societies as confirmatory tests to support the clinical diagnosis of brain death and to shorten otherwise necessary waiting periods of six to twelve hours. Most countries allow the use of EEG, which must demonstrate electrocortical silence over a certain period. Evoked cerebral potentials can demonstrate the successive loss of activity of various **afferent** pathways and are accepted in some countries as a confirmatory test. Other neurophysiological tests which demonstrate the loss of cerebral perfusion can be implemented. Brain **scintigraphy** can confirm the loss of isotope uptake into the brain. Doppler **sonography** also demonstrates cessation of brain perfusion.

While the concept of brain death remains widely accepted in the world, medical progress, clinical experience, social change, new methods of organ retrieval and unresolved conceptual issues have provided significant challenges to its early, almost unchallenged status. Even some of the states of the USA[25] have had to accept modifications. The State of New York, for example, adopted brain failure as a legal definition of death in 1987 and it has been difficult to override this claim. Nevertheless, one state (New Jersey) has passed legislation granting an exception to brain death on religious grounds. New York has not gone quite so far, but now recommends accommodation to such beliefs. The New York State Task Force on Life and the Law examined the question of objection to the brain death standard on religious or moral grounds, and recommended that "responses to individuals with religious or moral objections would best be addressed by health care facilities at the community level".

Although the vast majority of the countries of the globe have accepted brain-death criteria to determine death after failed resuscitation in respirator-dependent patients in deep coma, the debate on ethical, legal and conceptual grounds continues relentlessly. Concerning the use of ancillary tests, a group of authors emphasize that such tests are needed when the clinical criteria cannot be applied or when they are confounded. Ancillary tests include tests of intracranial blood circulation, electrophysiological tests, metabolic studies and tests for residual vagus nerve function (Young et al., 2006).[26]

An editorial in the British Medical Journal (Baumgartner and Gerstenbrand, 2002)[27] deals with the problems of hospitals without a neurologist. To verify brain-death criteria, the opinion of a neurologist, in some cases two, is required. This presents no problem in developed countries where usually there is one neurologist per 30,000 people. But a solution is needed for developing countries where there is perhaps only one neurologist per 3,000,000 population The authors believe that with simpler guidelines, non neurologists can be trained to follow the steps to verify that brain death has occurred.

We agree with this view. It is not the type of postgraduate medical training that makes the determination of death accurate; it is the accuracy of following the rules; the practice guidelines that were established by professional associations for the determination of brain death. Ethical, legal and conceptual matters concerning brain death are still argued, as is obvious from the Proceedings of the IV International Symposium on Coma and Death held in Havana. A selection of lectures, by authors who are prominent scholars in the field, was edited and published soon after the symposium (Machado and Shewmon, 2004).[28] As the editors state in the preface to their book "the motivation to ever deepen our knowledge about human death (and life) is a matter of human dignity".

Notes

1. Lazar, N. M., Shemie, S., Webster, G. C., Dickens B. M., Bioethics for clinicians: 24. Brain death, *CMAJ*, 20, (2001): 164.

2. Jennett, B., Brainstem death defines death in law, *BMJ*, 318, (1999): 1755. Jennett points out in this short note that a recent review by the Royal Colleges preferred the term brainstem death, but found that there was no need to modify the original diagnostic criteria outlined in 1976, which require two doctors to carry out specific tests on two occasions.

3. Kuchta, J., 55. Jahrestagung der Deutschen Gesellschaft für Neurochirurgie e.V. (DGNC), from Brain death versus brainstem death: An international analysis of historic and actual criteria to diagnose death <http://www.egms.de/en/meetings/dgnc2004/04dgnc0147.shtml>, accessed August 8, 2006.

4. Walker, E., Respirator brain, in id., *Cerebral Death* (Dallas: Professional Information Library, 1977): 114-118.

5. Pope Pius XII, The Prolongation of Life: Allocution to the International Congress of Anesthesiologists, November 24, 1957, in *The Pope Speaks,* Vol. 4, (1958): 393-398.

6. Definition of irreversible coma: Report of the Ad Hoc Committee of the Harvard Medical School to examine the definition of brain death, *JAMA,* 205, (1968): 337-340.

7. Skegg, P. D. G., The termination of artificial ventilation, in id., *Law Ethics and Medicine* (Oxford: Clarendon Press, 1984): 161-182.

8. Veatch, R. M., *Death, Dying and the Biological Revolution: Our last quest for responsibility*, rev. edn., (New Haven: Yale University Press, 1989).

9. Tooley, M., Decision to terminate life and the concept of person, in J. Ladd, (ed.), *Ethical Issues Relating to Life and Death* (New York: Oxford University Press, 1979): 62-93.

10. Ivan, L. P., Irreversible brain damage and related problems: Pronouncement of

death, *J Am Geriatr Soc,* 18, (1970): 816-822.

11. Ivan, L. P., Spinal reflexes in cerebral death, *Neurology,* 23, (1973): 650-652.

12. Baudouin, J. L., Criteria for determination of death: The approach of the Law Reform Commission of Canada, in T. P. Morley, (ed.), *Moral, Ethical, and Legal Issues in the Neurosciences* (Springfield, IL: Charles C. Thomas, 1981): 42-46.

13. Ivan, L. P., Time sequence in brain death in T. P. Morley, (ed.), *Moral, Ethical and Legal Issues in the Neurosciences* (Springfield, IL: Charles C. Thomas, 1981): 21-24.

14. Korein, J., Brain Death: Interrelated medical and social issues. Terminology, definitions, and usage, *Ann NY Acad Sci,* 315, (1978, Nov 17): 6-18.

15. Chagas, C., (ed.), *The Artificial Prolongation of Life and the Determination of the Exact Moment of Death* (Citta del Vaticano: Pontifica Academia Scientiarum, 1986).

16. Swash, M., Brain death: Still-unresolved issues worldwide, *Neurology,* 58,(2002): 9-10.

17. Wijdicks, E., Brain death worldwide: Accepted fact but no global consensus in diagnostic criteria, *Neurology,* 56, (2002): 20-25.

18. China's first brain death standard approved <http://www/china.org.cn/english/2004/May/94597.htm>, accessed May 28, 2006.

19. Jorgensen, E. O., Two standards of death in Denmark. Death in Denmark is either cardiac death or brain death. The 2nd International Symposium on Brain Death, Havana, Cuba, February 27-March 1, 1996 [abstract] <http://www.changesurfer.com/BD/1996/1996Abstracts.html>, accessed August 3, 2006.

20. Huet, H., Leroy, G., Toulas, P., et al., Radiological confirmation of brain death: Digitised cerebral parenchymography. Preliminary report, *Neuroradiology,* 38, (Suppl. I), (1996): S42-S46.

21. Sachedina, Abdulaziz, Brain Death in Islamic Jurisprudence <http://www.people.virginia.edu/~aas/article6.htm>, accessed June 28, 2006.

22. Thomke, F., Weilemam, L. S., Current concepts in diagnosing brain death in Germany [article in German], *Med Klin (Munich),* 95(2), (2000): 95-99.

23. Morioka, M., Reconsidering brain death: A lesson from Japan's fifteen years of experience, *Hastings Center Report,* 31, no. 4, (2001) <http://www.lifestufies.org/reconsidering.html>, accessed June 23, 2006.

24. Haupt, W. F., Rudolf, J., European Brain Death Codes: A Comparison of National Guidelines, *J Neurol,* 246(6), (1999): 432-437.

25. Freer, J., Ethics Committee Core Curriculum, Online Edition, Brain Death UB Center for Clinical Ethics and Humanities in Health Care <http://wings.buffalo. edu/faculty/research/bioethics/man-deth.html>, accessed August 24, 2006.

26. Young, B., Shemie, S., Doig, C., Teitelbaum, J., Brief review: The role of ancillary tests in the neurological determination of death, *CJA*, 53, (2006): 620-627.

27. Baumgartner, H., Gerstenbrand, F., Diagnosing brain death without a neurologist, *BMJ*, 324, (2002): 1471-1472.

28. Machado, G., Shewmon A. D., (eds.), *Brain Death and Disorders of Consciousness*, (New York: Kluwer Academic/Plenum Publishers, 2004).

CHAPTER 3
OTHER ISSUES RELATED TO DEATH

Discussion and disagreement should not discourage those who trust that the concept of brain death represents an important paradigm shift in the understanding of how and when human life ends. Nevertheless, as a result of some of the unsettled issues about brain death, ethical and legal dilemmas still surface at the bedside, in the courts and in the media. Sometimes it is religious orthodoxy, while at other times it is misunderstanding which fosters such disagreements. Such issues, some of them new, others older but still evolving, are presented in this chapter.

Dying with Dignity

Although most people would prefer to die at home, in modern society they often die in acute or chronic care hospitals due to serious illness or accident. It goes without saying that hospitals are unable to provide the privacy and warmth of the home environment. The patient is frequently disturbed for "vital signs", adjustments of equipment and various other routines. The general hubbub of activities make it almost impossible to rest and a patient's remaining life may be disordered and stressful instead of peaceful and calm.

In the 1960s, dying patients who did not fit into the usual active treatment pattern, were often moved into physical isolation for privacy, but this resulted in a kind of abandonment. Health care workers could see that a new, more compassionate approach was needed and new trends began to emerge such as the hospice concept (**palliative care**) and the "dying with dignity" movement.

The hospice concept and palliative care

The hospice movement, which began in Britain, was made known throughout the world by the work of Dr. Cicely Saunders,[1] who combined the caring skills with a pioneer program of pain control. She founded St. Christopher's Hospice, the world's first purpose-built hospice, in 1967. The hospice was founded on the principles of expert pain and symptom relief combined with holistic care to meet the physical, social, psychological and spiritual needs of patients and of their family and friends.

By the late 1980s there were 70 free-standing hospices in the UK. As of 1999, there were 175 independent hospices (Addington-Hall, 2005).[2] A hospice does not refer to a place of cure but rather to a haven of care which helps the gravely ill to have the best quality of life until they die. Highly skilled staff and volunteers enable the patient to be as free from pain as possible. Open discussion about fears and anxieties is encouraged and support is given to the patient's family, while involving them as much as possible in the patient's care. Even though a cure is not generally expected, healing and spiritual enrichment is still possible.

Compassionate care or palliative care and end-of-life support are now provided by many organizations throughout the world. The medical needs of a patient can vary widely depending on the disease, and palliative care can take place in a hospice, in the home or in hospitals. There are programs for common conditions such as cancer and AIDS and special care for those with chronic illness, such as dementia and coma. The National Hospice Foundation in the United States clearly states that it wishes to ensure ". . . that at the end of life, people should have the opportunity to maintain their dignity and self respect; live their final days pain-free; have the involvement and support of loved ones; and access the highest quality care available through hospice".[3]

As our life expectancy increases due to medical advances and healthier living, the number of elderly is expected to increase and the need for end-of-life care will increase.

In Canada, with its widely dispersed population, the hospice movement is embodied in Palliative Care Units. These units often exist as part of a large general hospital. In 1975 palliative care services within a hospital setting were introduced for the first time in North America by two Canadian hospitals: the St. Boniface Hospital in Winnipeg and the Royal Victoria Hospital in Montreal, for the management of patients suffering from terminal cancer. Bereavement counselling was provided by professionals or skilled volunteers and domiciliary care was extended to the home (Manning, 1984).[4] Canada now has 450 hospice palliative care programs.[5]

In 1981, the Palliative Care Foundation in Toronto, Ontario proposed a definition of palliative care. More than two decades later the definition is still pertinent:

> Palliative care is active compassionate care of the terminally ill at a time when they are no longer responsive to traditional treatment aimed at cure and prolongation of life and when the control of symptoms, physical and emotional, is paramount. It is multidisciplinary in its approach and encompasses the patient, the family and the community in its scope.

That same year, the Department of Health and Welfare Canada sought to develop national practices in palliative care with the publication of the "Palliative Care Services Guidelines" and, in 1983, the first university institute for research and education on palliative care was created at the University of Ottawa.

The Canadian Hospice Palliative Care Association is a national, charitable, non-profit association whose mission is to provide leadership in hospice palliative care, and to advocate for increased programs and services. According to this association, only 15%

of Canadians have access to palliative care either in their home or in a hospice. Of the 220,000 Canadians who die each year, 75% die in acute-care hospitals or long-term care facilities. To deliver palliative care in an acute-care hospital stretches both the hospital and provincial health-care budget to the limit. This is not the best use of health-care facilities. Acute-care hospitals are focused on saving lives while palliative care is concerned with the last stages of life; to live with dignity and without pain for as long as life lasts.

As stated by the World Health Organization[6] in their definition of palliative care:

> Palliative care is an approach which improves the quality of life of patients and their families facing life-threatening illness, through the prevention, assessment and treatment of pain and other physical, psychosocial and spiritual problems.

There is worldwide interest in hospice or palliative care expansion and implementation. There are national associations in almost every European country as listed by the European Association for Palliative Care.[7] Associations also extend to the nation members of the World Health Organization and the United States has several established organizations such as the National Hospice Foundation.[8]

There are many papers in the medical literature in support of the advantages of palliative care; we cite only a few from the large number available. (Steinhauser, 2000),[9] (Sabatowski, 2001),[10] (Lloyd-Williams, 2004)[11] There are also many excellent websites and books on research, education, standards of development and different approaches throughout the global community. There is a universal interest in seeking an end to life that protects individual dignity, provides freedom from pain and encourages the love and comfort that comes from friends and family.

The "right to die" movement and assisted suicide

Advances in medical knowledge and technology have enabled life to be prolonged, but may also prolong suffering. The concept of alleviating suffering is different from that of the hospice movement and it was pioneered by a movement and association called the World Federation of Right to Die Societies.

In Canada it is called Dying With Dignity (DWD), a registered charitable organization whose mission is to improve the quality of dying for all Canadians in accordance with their own wishes, values, and beliefs.

To accomplish this, DWD:

[would] inform and educate individuals about their rights to determine and choose health care options at the end of life; build public support for legal change to permit voluntary, physician-assisted dying; work toward the legal recognition of health-care directives across Canada.

[would provide] Living Wills, Enduring Powers of Attorney for Personal Care and other advance health care directives and counselling and advocacy services to members, upon request; information, referral and support to individuals making important end-of-life decisions; educational materials and access to their resource library; speakers for meetings on a variety of topics; a national, quarterly newsletter.

DWD initiates and participates in public forums, is a leading information source for the media, and is a reliable source of specialized information and educational materials. Established in 1980, "Dying With Dignity" is a member of the World Federation of Right to Die Societies that represents 38 organizations from 23 different countries. Since one of the primary aims of this association is to promote the right to die by means of assisted suicide, the scope of this issue will be further detailed in Chapter Six, which focuses on euthanasia.

Public opinion confirms that the majority of Americans worry about pain during the dying process and that they fear living in a "vegetable" state. In 1997, Gallup's "Spiritual Beliefs and the Dying Process" survey (Blizzard, 2002)[12] found that 73% of American adults fear "the possibility of being vegetable-like for some period of time" before their deaths, and 67% fear "the possibility of great physical pain" before death. Such concerns have introduced a grey ethical area regarding what the medical community should and should not do to promote the continuation of life, and how to ensure patients' rights to maintain dignity in death. It is an area that will only grow thornier as researchers develop new ways to extend life using stem cells and cloned organs.

In 2001, the Governor of New York State constituted a Task Force on Life and the Law that will also be discussed in the chapter on euthanasia (Pataki, 2001).[13]

The patient's rights

In addition to the generalities that are laid out in various charters of rights (the right to freedom, life, and happiness), patients have, and always have had rights, under the law. This applies to the special circumstances under which an individual enters a hospital, or engages a physician in a contractual bind to diagnose and treat an illness to the best of his or her ability, and according to the proper standards of medicine. Patients have the right of protection against professional negligence, the right to explanation of treatments and the right to refuse a recommended treatment. Most hospitals have adopted a code of ethics which lists the rights of a patient, whether adult or child.

In the context of death and dying, there are certain rights which usually centre around such issues as the right to die, the right to refuse treatment, the living will, beneficent euthanasia and similar difficult matters that involve not only ethical but also legal considerations. Because all of these issues are important, they will be discussed under separate headings. In this section only the rights related to making decisions in general, such as the consent or refusal of treatment and difficulties associated with the incompetence of the patient (children, mentally disturbed individuals, and the patient in coma) will be discussed. Books on ethical and legal issues relevant to the patient's rights are listed in the notes, (Ladd, 1979),[14] (Veatch, 1989),[15] (Skegg, 1984)[16] and (Meyers, 1970).[17]

In technologically advanced societies, the majority of people die in hospitals or in nursing homes where basic human rights for the terminally ill are assured. Because of advanced cardiac and trauma life support, a significant number of patients are in coma or in a critical condition and unable to make decisions for themselves. Decision-making is often a medical emergency and involves the consent of a relative. While the law makes clear provisions about consent, it is for the most part the ethical principles of physicians and surgeons that can ensure basic human rights for terminally or critically ill patients.

It is the legal right of every mentally competent adult to refuse life-sustaining treatment. This right is never questioned while the patient is treated at home or in an outpatient programme (e.g. kidney dialysis). However, in a hospital setting, this right may be in conflict with the duty of the hospital staff to provide the best professional care.

Physicians who treat their patients without consent are guilty of assault or battery. A doctor can be held liable in a legal action if the consent to treatment has not been an "informed consent". Informed consent must include the knowledge of the terminal nature of an illness, and in the case of coma, the consenting relative must be aware of the risks of a procedure and the chances of survival when extraordinary measures are used to save or prolong life.

The terminally ill patient has the right to choose his or her place of death. Unfortunately, nursing homes have become the dumping ground of the aged and if there is no place to die at home, some terminally ill persons are subject to inhuman conditions and much indignity.

The hospice movement, which at present is reserved for the care of patients for whom management of pain is the primary concern, could be used as a model for all dying persons, making it possible to draw the family and the dying patients closer together.

The Canadian patient's rights are available in book form, (Rozovsky, 1994).[18] In the context of dying and death, the author discusses the Right to Die, The Right to Refuse Care and the Living Will, and emphasizes that:

- The law does not tell doctors when the diagnosis of death is to be made.
- The diagnosis of death is important because various legal rights of the deceased end, and various legal rights and duties of others may arise as a result of wills, insurance, contracts and legislation.
- There is no legal right to die, though there is a right to refuse care or treatment even though it may result in death.
- There is a right to live, but not to require doctors and hospitals to provide unreasonable or unavailable care or treatment in order to sustain life.

A wealth of information is available from a recently published book (Blank and Merrick, 2005).[19] The book presents an in-depth study by several authors, who discuss end-of-life decisions in Brazil, China, Germany, India, Israel, Japan, Kenya, the Netherlands, Taiwan, Turkey, the United Kingdom and the United States of America.

Not surprisingly, the how, where and why of dying, show extreme variability, which depends partly on the cultural and partly on the economic diversity of the selected countries. Of all the countries studied in the book, only Japan, Taiwan, the United Kingdom and the United States systematically collect data on death. In the majority of the studied countries, most people die at home, but in the Western countries more patients reach life's end elsewhere. The United Kingdom and the United States have the highest rates of in-hospital deaths. In the USA, 55% of deaths occur in hospitals, 25% at home, 9% in nursing homes, 9% in hospices, and 1% in other places. In the UK 65% of deaths occur in hospitals, 20% at home, 4% in hospices, and 8% in other communal establishments. In Germany about half of the deaths occur in hospitals.

It is, of course, the patient's right to expect dignity and respect while in end-of-life care. As a recent study of seriously ill patients shows (Hyland et al., 2006)[20] the most important matters for end-of-life decisions were "not to be kept alive on life support when there is little hope for meaningful recovery" (55.7% of respondents), followed by "trust and confidence in the doctors looking after you" (55%) and that "information about the disease be communicated by the doctor in an honest manner" (44.1%). It was also very important "to complete things and prepare for life's end–life review, resolving conflicts, saying goodbye" (43.9%).

The doctor's obligation

The doctor, according to the Hippocratic Oath and other ethical and professional commitments, has a variety of obligations towards the dying person. To relieve suffering without shortening life, to ensure the spiritual needs of the patient and to maintain a close, human doctor-patient relationship are inherent good medical practices. The patient may have a number of questions which are sometimes difficult to answer. Nevertheless, these questions have to be answered with honesty and compassion.

The most common problem is how much to tell the patient. Relatives frequently suggest that the patient should not know that he or she is going to die. Interestingly, the majority of patients never ask about the time of their death and whether or not their illness is fatal. If the question is asked, it is the doctor's obligation to tell the truth. But when it comes to the question of, "How much time do I have left?", the uncertainty of the time removes the obligation to give dates or even guess at the remaining time, since the answer can only be given in vague terms. The statistical spread in predicting survival is so great that even with the common fatal diseases, the margin of error can be weeks, months or even years.

Imminent death is another matter. In the vast majority of cases when death is imminent, the patient is so unwell that the question does not arise because the patient is preoccupied with the relief of pain or other forms of intense suffering. In other instances of imminent death, the patient may be in a coma and the question would come from the relatives. Doctors have an obligation only to inform the nearest relative who should, in turn, give the news to the rest of the family. Sometimes the whole family sits together in a "quiet room" or in the doctor's office wanting to hear the grave news collectively. If this form of communication is chosen by the nearest relative, the doctor is obliged to consult collectively with all members of the family.

An important question is that of pain relief, which is the greatest problem for the sufferer of an incurable disease, most often cancer. When cancer spreads into various parts of the body, particularly into bones and in the vicinity of nerve roots or peripheral nerves, the condition becomes extremely painful. Many times, when pain control is a serious problem, the illness has already reached a terminal stage and the question of passive euthanasia and the "no resuscitation" order may have to be addressed by the members of a health care team.

The Canadian Medical Association summarizes the relevant passages this way: [21]

- Respect the right of a competent patient to accept or reject any medical care recommended.
- Respect your patient's reasonable request for a second opinion from a physician of the patient's choice.
- Ascertain whenever possible and recognize the patient's wishes about the initiation, continuation or cessation of life-sustaining treatment.
- Respect the intentions of an incompetent patient as they were expressed (e.g. through a valid advance directive or proxy designation) before the patient became incompetent.
- When the intentions of an incompetent patient are unknown and when no formal mechanism for making treatment decisions is in place, render such treatment as you believe to be in accordance with the patient's values or, if these are unknown, the patient's best interest.
- Be considerate of the patient's family and significant others and cooperate with them in the patient's interest.

The "Do not resuscitate" order

It is the patient's right not to be subject to undue prolongation of useless suffering and it is the doctor's obligation to relieve suffering. The patient has the right to refuse treatment even to his own detriment, and when the patient has made an advance directive or a living will, it is the doctor's obligation to consider the wishes of the patient who is terminally ill. It may be the patient's wish that resuscitative measures are not to be used if a cardiac arrest occurs. There are three forms of advance directives: (1) living will, (2) durable power of attorney for health care and (3) oral statements.

In 1891, the US Supreme Court mandated that no right is more sacred than guarding one's person and, thus, one's autonomy. American courts recognize a competent adult's right to refuse health-care treatment even if the withholding of such treatment could result in the patient's death. The more difficult cases have arisen when the patient is incompetent.

Unfortunately several studies in the USA have shown that advance directives are often ignored. Goodman and colleagues (Goodman et al., 1998)[22] reviewed the medical records of 401 patients over the age of 65 years admitted to the ICU (Intensive Care Unit) between 1992 and 1995. Only 5% had an advance directive. Of the patients with advance directives who died, 40% received CPR despite pre-existing instructions to forgo this procedure. In this study, the presence of an advance directive did not influence care or ICU length of stay.

A survey of 1,832 patients in five tertiary care hospitals showed that only 23% of seriously ill hospitalized patients had discussed preferences for CPR with their physician. Of those patients who had not discussed end-of-life issues, 58% were not even interested in doing so (Hoffmann, 1997).[23]

On the other hand, it is becoming a common practice in hospitals to issue an order not to resuscitate. This is done by the attending physician only after careful deliberation with the relatives and the health care team. Emergency procedures such as the repeated resuscitation of a patient suffering from a terminal disease are often considered to be excessive by both relatives and medical personnel. If, in the case of vegetative survival, an overwhelming complication develops which could claim the patient's life without suffering, the patient may be allowed to die. In another instance, an order not to resuscitate may be written when resuscitation from a cardiac arrest would only lead to several repeated instances of "dying" from respiratory or cardiac failure, and prolong suffering and dying. This situation also creates problems as reported by Asch and colleagues.[24] A survey of 879 physicians in adult ICUs evaluated their practices with regard to withholding and withdrawing life support. Almost all respondents (96%) said they had withheld or withdrawn life-sustaining therapy and most did so frequently. Many physicians unilaterally withheld (83%), or withdrew (82%), treatment they considered medically futile. Some physicians (34%) continued treatment even though patients or surrogates requested that therapy be stopped. Physicians cited the following reasons for continuing life support despite patient or surrogate requests to stop:

1. Belief that the patient had a reasonable chance of recovery (77%)
2. Belief that the family may not be acting in the patient's best interest (39%) and
3. Fear of malpractice (19%).

In Canada, there have been many discussions between nurses, doctors, lawyers and administrators about the ethical and legal implications of the no resuscitation order. Initially, this order was given by a physician to a nurse verbally since it was felt that it was unethical to write such an order. With the increasing number of malpractice lawsuits, doctors began to worry about the legal consequences and this made them even more inclined to avoid a written order. Since, however, it is usually the nurse who witnesses cardiac arrest, the ethical burden falls upon the nursing profession, not only with legal overtones but in conflict with their own professional and ethical standards and individual convictions.

The Canadian Medical Association's doctor's code of ethics with respect to dying patients states that an ethical physician:

will allow death to occur with dignity and comfort when death of the body appears inevitable

may support the body when clinical death of the brain has occurred, but need not prolong life by unusual or heroic means.

From this code of ethics the "do not resuscitate policy" evolved. This policy was discussed extensively by a Committee at McMaster University, Hamilton, Canada. It became a matter of reference at the eighth World Congress of the Federation of Neurological Surgeons in Toronto in July 1985 at the meeting of the Federation's Legal and Ethical Committee. The senior author of this book was a member of the Committee that presented the following draft for discussion.

When a "Do Not Resuscitate" order is considered, the following guidelines may be useful:

1. If the patient is competent:
The relevant facts shall be discussed with the patient and his choice should be known. The implementation of his choice is the doctor's responsibility. If the patient does not wish unusual treatment, the Do Not Resuscitate (**DNR**) order shall be written in the chart by the attending physician along with a detailed note in the chart concerning the discussion with the patient.
The DNR order shall be reassessed from time to time. The patient may request the removal of the DNR at any time. If the reasons or facts for the DNR order change, a temporary removal of the order shall be made by the physician until the situation is discussed again with the patient and a new decision can be reached.
2. If the patient is incompetent:
The above policy as it applies to mentally ill or unconscious patients and sometimes to children under sixteen years of age is only implemented with the involvement and consent of the nearest relative or guardian.
3. Reasons and relevant facts to consider for a DNR order:
Reasonable estimates by the attending physician about the following:

a) the irreversibility of the patient's condition or the irreparability of damage

b) the length of time the patient may live with and without intervention

c) the quality of life (intense suffering) versus the short term gain of time (patient in coma, or under the heaviest sedation to cope with pain and suffering).

4. Documentation:

All "do not resuscitate" orders should be written on the physician's order sheet and signed by the attending physician. All relevant facts should be noted in the progress notes of the patient's medical record and discussed with the health care team (resident, head nurse, social worker) involved in the patient's management. The relevant facts should be reviewed by the attending physician at reasonable intervals and noted in the patient's chart.

These early attempts to define the "do not resuscitate" order as an acceptable hospital policy have gone through many refinements and there are several variations from one hospital to another.

The Living Will

The *Oxford Dictionary* provides the following definition:

a written statement detailing a person's desires regarding their medical treatment in circumstances in which they are no longer able to express informed consent.[25]

There are several alternative forms and names for a Living Will, such as the "Durable Medical Power of Attorney" and the "Advance Medical Directive". They allow people to state what they want for their own medical care if they are unable to make decisions for themselves. You can:

1. Direct that a specific procedure or treatment be provided,

such as artificially administered hydration (fluids) or nutrition (feeding);

2. Direct that a specific procedure or treatment be withheld; or

3. Appoint a person to act as your agent in making health care decisions for you, if it is determined that you are unable to make health care decisions for yourself. This includes the decision to make anatomical gifts of a specific part or parts of your body via organ and tissue donation, or of all of your body.

A Living Will allows a person to convey his or her wishes regarding treatment when those wishes can no longer be personally communicated.

A Medical Power of Attorney allows a person to designate someone to make health-care decisions for them when the person is unable.

California passed the first "right-to-die" law in 1976 and as of 1985 at least twenty-five states had similar or identical laws. The need for this kind of legislation developed from two contributing factors. On the one hand, the pressure of technology compels doctors to prolong life with extraordinary means in all cases, for fear of prosecution arising from the malpractice crisis in the United States. On the other hand, patients also have fears arising from this same technology and do not want to be caught in senseless prolongation of life and agony by artificial maintenance, if restoration of health is not possible.

From these justified concerns, the concept of "living will" developed. The living will expresses the wishes of an individual to members of the family, doctors or clergymen, in an informal way, about the use of extraordinary means when death is unavoidable. Because of further concerns about the legality or applicability of such wishes, more and more individuals sign statements known by a variety of names. The best known of these documents is called "A Living Will". Distributed by the Euthanasia Educational Council, it was first published in 1969. Its central paragraph reads:

Death is as much a reality as birth, growth, maturity and old age—it is the only certainty of life. If the time comes when I__
____, can no longer take part in decisions for my own future,

let this statement stand as an expression of my wishes, while I am still of sound mind.

If the situation should arise in which there is no reasonable expectation of my recovery from physical or mental disability, I request that I be allowed to die and not be kept alive by artificial means or "heroic measures". I do not fear death itself as much as the indignities of deterioration, dependence, and hopeless pain. I, therefore, ask that medication be mercifully administered to me to alleviate suffering even though this may hasten the moment of death.

To date, millions of Living Wills have been distributed. Although not legally binding, they do assert to family members and health professionals how a person chooses to die.

Notes

1. Saunders, Dame Cicely (1918-2005). English philanthropist, founder of the hospice movement, which aims to provide a caring and comfortable environment in which people with terminal illnesses can die. She was the medical director of St Christopher's Hospice in Sydenham, South London, 1967-85, and later became its chair. She wrote *Care of the Dying* (1960) and edited several books on death and dying and hospice care.

2. Addington-Hall, J. M., Karlsen, S., A national survey of health professionals and volunteers working in voluntary hospices in the UK, II, *Palliat Med*, 19(1), (2005): 49-57.

3. <http://www.nationalhospicefoundation.org/templates/1/index.cfm>, accessed May 27, 2006.

4. Manning, M., *The Hospice Alternative* (London: Souvenir Press, 1984).

The author gives a comprehensive survey of the hospice movement worldwide with special reference to the UK and Canada.

5. <http://www.stjoe.on.ca/svc_pall_care_canada.html>, accessed May 27, 2006.

6. <http://www.who.int/hiv/topics/palliative/care/en/index1.html>, accessed May 27, 2006.

7. <http://eapcnet.org/organisations/asseurope.html>, accessed May 26, 2006.

8. <http://nationalhospicefoundation.org>, accessed September 06, 2006.

9. Steinhauser, K. E., Christakis, N., Clipp, E., et al., Factors considered important at the end of life by patients, family, physicians, and other care providers, *JAMA*, 284, (2000): 2476-2482.

10. Sabatowski, R., Radbruch, L., Nauck, F., et al., Development and state of the in-patient palliative care institutions in Germany, *Schmerz*, 15, (2001): 312-319.

11. Lloyd-Williams, M., MacLeod, R. D., A systematic review of teaching and learning in palliative care within the medical undergraduate curriculum, *Med Teach*, 26, (2004): 683-690.

12. Blizzard, R., The Gallup Poll "Right to Die or Dead to Rights?", (June 5, 2002) <http://poll.gallup.com/content/default.aspx?ci=6265&pg=1>, accessed August 15, 2006.

13. Pataki, Governor George, New York State Task Force on Life and the Law, 2001 <http://health.state.ny.us/nysdoh/consumer/patient/chap5.html>, accessed April 30, 2006.

14. Ladd, J., (ed.), *Ethical Issues Relating to Life and Death* (New York: Oxford University Press, 1979): 118-145.

15. Veatch, R. M., (ed.), *Death, Dying and the Biological Revolution: Our last quest for responsibility*, rev. edn., (New Haven: Yale University Press, 1989).

16. Skegg, P. D. G., *Law, Ethics, and Medicine* (Oxford: Clarendon Press, 1984): 75-98.

17. Meyers, D., *The Human Body and the Law: A medico-legal study* (Chicago: Aldine Publishing Company, 1970): 139-154.

18. Rozovsky, L., *The Canadian Patient's Book of Rights*, rev. edn., (Toronto: Doubleday, 1994): 201-209.

19. Blank, R. H., Merrick J. C., (eds.), *End-of-Life Decision Making: A cross-national study* (Cambridge, MA: MIT Press, 2005).

20. Hyland, D. K., Dodek, P., Rocker, G., et al., What matters most in end-of-life care: perceptions of seriously ill patients and their family members, *CMAJ*, 174(5), (2006): 627-633.

21. Permission to quote was granted by the Canadian Medical Association.

22. Goodman, M. D., Tarnoff, M., Slotman, G. J., Effect of advance directives on the management of elderly critically ill patients, *Crit Care Med*, 26, (1998): 701-704.

23. Hoffmann, J. C., Wenger, N. S., Davis, R. B., et al., Patient preferences for communication with physicians about end-of-life decisions, *Ann Intern Med*, 127, (1997): 1-12.

24. Asch, D. A., Hansen-Flaschen, J., Lanken, P. N., Decision to limit or continue life-sustaining treatment by critical care physicians in the United States: Conflicts between physician's practices and patient wishes, *Am J Respir Crit Care Med*, 151, (1995): 288-292.

25. *Oxford Concise Dictionary* (Oxford: Oxford University Press, 2006).

CHAPTER 4
ORGAN TRANSPLANTATION AND THE TIME SEQUENCE IN BRAIN DEATH

We have learned to see death in slow motion and to understand that the "moment of death" can be a time-consuming diagnostic procedure at the end of which doctors must agree that death has occurred. The flowchart below (Fig. 4) shows the path from the state of coma to a possible recovery or brain death. If respiratory support is stopped, cardiac arrest would follow in minutes and by progressive cellular death, through **autolysis** and decay, the body would reach complete organic death.

If, on the other hand, organ transplantation is considered, intensive care of the body will continue with respiratory and other necessary support to maintain tissue oxygenation. After certifying death by the use of brain-oriented criteria, which for logistical reasons may take several hours, or more, the transplant team takes custody of the body until the donated organs are removed in the operating room. The removal requires sterile conditions like any other operative procedure. When the transplant surgeon or surgeons complete their work, respiratory support will stop and in a few minutes cardiac arrest will follow. The time of irreversible apnea—brain arrest—ends here and progressive cellular death continues in the remaining organs of the body as would have happened without the use of the respirator.

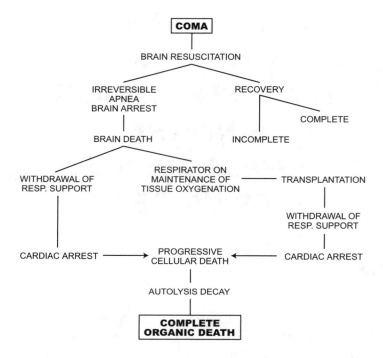

Fig. 4. *This flowchart shows possible sequential events from a comatose state to a successful or failed resuscitation. If brain death is declared and organ donation is considered, the respiratory support will continue to maintain heartbeat and tissue oxygenation until the removal of the donated organs is completed.*

This diagram also presents certain terms that refer to the various stages of dying and assigns the "moment" of death to a time segment which follows the failed attempt of brain resuscitation.

Thus, the time of death shifts from the absence of respiration and heartbeat to a time when death coexists with the artificially maintained viability of the other organs of the body. Had the respirator not been turned on, the heart would have stopped and tissue cellular death would have occurred in all the other organs of the body.

The death of the brain in apnoeic coma is ascertained by two health professionals (usually a neurologist and a neurosurgeon or an intensivist) who are qualified to make this diagnosis. The attending physician, who must be guided by professional ethics and the law, will enter the time when the diagnosis confirmed that brain death has occurred and notes whether the respirator was turned off or the body transferred to the transplant team for continued support and removal of the donated organs.

The extreme care taken in the development of new guidelines for the declaration of death was exemplified by the Memorandum issued by the Conference of Medical Royal Colleges and their Faculties in the United Kingdom (Appendix B), in the President's Commission in the USA and in the Law Reform Commission in Canada as discussed previously. It has taken several years of consultation by a large number of experts to produce these important documents. Yet some confusion still exists, even among health professionals, when the management of a brain-dead patient becomes a task at the bedside or a topic of discussion in a variety of forums (classrooms, meetings, publications).

Some people still believe that the withdrawal of artificial support in brain death is the same as active euthanasia (Byrne et al., 2005).[1] Quoting Pope Pius XII, the authors state:

> The death of the person is a single event, consisting in the total disintegration of that unitary and integrated whole that is the personal self. It results from the separation of the life-principle (or soul) from the corporal reality of the person. Pope Pius XII declared this same truth when he stated that human life continues when its vital functions manifest themselves even with the help of artificial processes.

However, they fail to add Pope Pius' statement in totality. The original text of the Pope is cited below.[2]

> It remains for the doctor, and especially the anesthesiologist, to give a clear and precise definition of "death" and the "moment of death" of a patient who passes away in a state of unconsciousness. Here one can accept the usual concept of complete and final separation of the soul from the body; but in

practice one must take into account the lack of precision of the terms "body" and "separation".

Discussing the continuation or discontinuation of respiratory support Pope Pius XII stated:

> . . . since these forms of treatment go beyond the ordinary means to which one is bound, it cannot be held that there is an obligation to use them nor, consequently, that one is bound to give the doctor permission to use them.

Others may think that continuation of artificial support would result in survival and should be maintained even if it ends in a vegetative state. Neither of these assumptions is true, although in a few cases, for example, in order to support the life of a fetus in the case of a pregnant woman, artificial maintenance has been continued as long as possible.

The flowchart of the stages of coma deserves careful study in order to understand the various pathophysiological changes following an acute insult to the brain which could lead to recovery (with or without disability) or death.

Coma, in many cases, is a transient state of abnormal function of the brain. Through various measures that we have already discussed under brain resuscitation, complete recovery is a possible outcome. On the other hand, if brain resuscitation has failed, the final common pathway to death is **brain swelling** and compression of the lower brainstem exactly where the respiratory centre is located. This is why unresponsive coma, absence of brainstem reflexes (pupillary response to light, blinking after touching the cornea, eye movement after **caloric stimulation** of the ear canal) and prolonged absence of spontaneous respiration are the basic signs proving that the brain is dead.

If we consider that the only outlet from the skull is at the level of the lower brainstem and the respiratory centre (see Fig. 1 on page 34), it becomes easy to understand why damage to this area from increased pressure and brain herniation represent the final common pathway to irreversible coma.

How does this occur? Lack of oxygen, infection, brain hemorrhage or severe head injury would first cause swelling of the tissues inside the skull. An increase in volume inside a closed container causes high pressure. In the case of the skull the intracranial pressure will rise but compensation can occur when spinal fluid shifts out of the cavity into the spinal subarachnoid spaces through the **foramen magnum**, an opening at the base of the skull where the lower brainstem, the **medulla oblongata**, joins the spinal cord.

As the intracranial pressure reaches a higher level and the liquid contents from the skull (venous blood and **CSF**) are essentially squeezed out of the cranial cavity, the pressure will shift brain tissue towards the foramen magnum, the only outlet from the skull. Compression of the small arteries will interfere with oxygen supply to the nerve cells and confusion, somnolence or coma may develop. As the pressure keeps increasing, more brain tissue will be shifted towards the foramen magnum. The medical term for this pathological entity is **foraminal herniation**, a clinical emergency when certain signs and symptoms clearly signal to the trained health professional that the respiratory centre is compromised and the patient may stop breathing. Brain resuscitation could reverse the condition, but when the pressure inside the skull reaches the level of the mean arterial blood pressure, the flow of oxygenated blood to the brain will stop and the oxygen-starved nerve cells both in the brainstem and the higher centres (in the midbrain, **thalamus** and the cortex) begin to die. If countermeasures don't occur in time, damage to the nerve cells becomes irreversible and neither spontaneous breathing nor higher functions of the brain can return when all the nerve cells have died. Since the 1960s we have called this condition, rightly or wrongly, "brain death".

The diagnostic method for determining brain death is an elaborate process logistically. It requires repeated neurological assessments, EEG examinations, consultation and sometimes other ancillary tests (measurement of cerebral blood flow, angiogram etc.). The time-frame between the failed treatment (i.e., the inability to resuscitate the brain) and the suspicion of irreversible brain damage, and proof of brain death can be lengthy–hours or even days. This time-frame can be referred to as the time of irreversible apnea (brain death). Mechanical ventilation would continue pending the fulfilment of medical, legal and/or ethical criteria of brain death or simply, death. Brain death, if we think of it as an "irreversible brain failure when resuscitation is no longer possible", is not only a lack of functional capacity, it also means that the brain tissue is irreversibly dead and the other organs' viability is artificial, maintained only by a mechanical device, the respirator.

It may be helpful to remember that even with the old criteria of death (absence of respiration and heartbeat), it was the state of nerve cells in the brainstem that made "death" reversible, or irreversibly final. Before the invention of respirators, repeated manual compression of the chest was used to maintain oxygenation of the body. If spontaneous breathing did not return and the pupils were dilated, manual respiration was stopped after 20-30 minutes and the patient was declared dead.

The fact that many patients on the respirator (using conventional criteria) were already dead, led to the term "beating-heart cadaver", the concept of "brain death" and the need to redefine death. Since the moment of brain death cannot be established without prolonged diagnostic procedures and consultation, it remains a matter of debate, but accepted by most, that the time of death should be the time when the verification of brain death becomes complete. This time of agreement may of course be hours or days after the biological time of death.

The time of biological death is irrelevant from the standpoint of management because medical ethics require that the attending physician provides optimum medical care until the diagnosis of death is firmly established. The courts, on the other hand, in the case of a lawsuit concerning inheritance, may insist on pinpointing the time of biological death, which may have occurred a few hours or even days prior to the confirmed diagnosis of brain death. The most recent Canadian guidelines (Shemie et al., 2006) is an excellent document which states that the legal time of death is the first declaration of brain death.[3]

Upon agreement that death has occurred, the attending physician enters it into the patient's record as the "time of death". From that moment, one of two courses of action is possible. If no transplantation is considered, the attending physician terminates artificial support of the body by turning off the respirator. The heart will keep beating for a few minutes, until all remaining oxygen is used up by the organs and the lack of oxygen stops all those cells in the heart which trigger heartbeat. Cardiac arrest will follow in about 8-20 minutes and should be charted as the "time of asystole" which simply means the time when the heart stopped beating.

If, on the other hand, organ transplantation is planned, the attending physician transfers the body into the custody of the transplant team, under the care of another physician. Mechanical ventilation is continued while a host of laboratory tests are performed to secure ideal organ donor management. The time interval between death and transplantation can be called the time of artificial maintenance of tissue oxygenation. After the surgical removal of organs, the mechanical respirator is turned off and asystole will occur within 8-20 minutes.

Talking with the patient's family about these stages with tactful gentleness and as much clarity as possible, helps to eliminate unwelcome anxiety at a time when confusion may add emotional burden to the grief of relatives and to the mental strain of the professional team.

Death is a gradual process as is the declaration of cerebral death, brain death, or brainstem death. The argument by ethicists, physicians and lawyers continues as to how to name these brain-oriented criteria and whether or not the concept of death is confused with its criteria. And, although the Uniform Determination of Death Act, for example, is accepted by all states in the United States of America, there are minor refinements and differences from one hospital to another. The attempt to fine-tune protocols does not mean that the concept and the criteria of brain death are invalid; nevertheless, it would simplify matters if uniform, national practice standards could be achieved in all countries.

Organ donation and transplantation protocols

An editorial in the *New England Journal of Medicine* (Capron, 2001)[4] aptly characterized the legal and ethical problems around the determination of death:

> If one subject in health law and bioethics can be said to be at once well settled and persistently unresolved, it is how to determine that death has occurred. Once this determination involved simply the measurement of vital signs. It was as often performed by laypersons as by physicians. Now it is often a complex matter requiring specialized expertise and raising both conceptual and practical difficulties.

These issues are reasonably well settled for those who often see brain-dead patients, but not so with those who are in charge of the maintenance of the body and who do the removal of the organs. This may be the reason for the frequent renewal of practice guidelines. A summary of excellent suggestions appears in a recent issue of the **CMA** Journal (Shemie et al., 2006).[5]

With advances in medical technology and **immunosuppressive therapy** (particularly the advent of cyclosporine), organ transplantation is now an acceptable alternative to other forms of treatment (hemodialysis, peritoneal dialysis, artificial heart assist), or no treatment at all. Treatment of a number of end-stage diseases that involve the kidneys, heart and liver are increasingly successful and corneal grafting restores vision in those with scarred or diseased corneal tissue. Today, the main limiting factor to the further development of the science and practice of transplantation is the available supply of donor organs and tissues.

In Canada alone (source Health and Welfare Canada, workshop held on October 3-4, 1984 Ottawa, Ontario) approximately 1,000 patients awaited donated kidneys and an estimated 600 corneal transplants were needed. More than twenty years later the problem persists and the list of desperate patients waiting for organ donation has grown considerably. An estimation of the number of potential donors revealed some surprising figures (Sheehy et al., 2003).[6] They found that in 1999 the number of potential donors in their study was 5,462, yet the number of actual donors in the same year was only 2,399.

As a group of transplant specialists recently claimed (Wood et al., 2004)[6] "even in the face of the urgent need for transplantable organs, there continues to be a disparity between the number of potential organ donors and that of actual donors." They suggest that reducing this disparity requires the early retrieval of organs that offer the greatest likelihood of successful outcomes for the recipients. This strategy depends on the optimal care of the potential donors even after brain death has occurred.

To understand the effort made by dedicated professionals to save a person's life and when the outcome is unsuccessful, how the death of that person may save another life, it might be useful to retrace the sequence from brain injury to transplantation. These connected events were well summarized in the Canadian Medical Association Journal (Shemie et al., 2003):[8]

> The sequence initiated by devastating brain injury may include (1) resuscitation in the field, (2) evaluation and stabilization in the emergency department, (3) referral and access to ICU services, (4) prognostication, (5) ICU-based neuroprotective therapies, (6) withholding or withdrawal of life support, (7) outcomes including survival, death by cardiopulmonary criteria or death by neurological determination and (8) optimal end-of-life care, including tissue and organ donation.

It is obvious from this sequence that the logistics of organ transplantation is a multi-factorial, complex activity. It requires optimum performance that will equally help the survival of the victim as well as contribute to a higher proportion of organ donations, to offset the existing negative balance between brain death and donation of organs.

In spite of the unresolved and debated issues about brain death and transplantation, both the concept and the practice have gained acceptance in most parts of the world. Transplantation of organs from both living and deceased donors has produced a major advance in treating patients with fatal or debilitating conditions. Table IV shows the number of organ transplantations in the USA during the first two months of the year 2006.

Table IV

TRANSPLANTS PERFORMED JANUARY-FEBRUARY 2006 USA

Total	4,508
Deceased donor	3,391
Living donor	1,112

Table V (based on **OPTN** data, 05/26/2006) shows the numbers of those waiting for the donation of one or two organs. The waiting list for kidneys is twice as long as all the others together. A mitigating factor is that the kidney is a paired organ and that viable kidneys can be obtained from deceased donors.

Table V

WAITING LIST OF CANDIDATES AS OF JUNE 6, 2006 USA

All	92,256
Kidney	66,820
Pancreas	1,740
Kidney/Pancreas	2,480
Intestine	222
Heart	2,959
Lung	3,001
Heart/Lung	147

Table VI shows the National Database statistics of transplanted organs in the UK.

Table VI

IN THE UK BETWEEN 1 APRIL 2005 AND 31 MARCH 2006:

Organs from 765 people who died were used to save or dramatically improve many people's lives through 2,196 transplants. The total includes 126 non-heartbeating donors, 43% more than the previous year.

A total of 1,799 patients received a kidney transplant of which 594 (33%) were given their kidney by a friend or relative–this increase of 25% sets another record for the number of living kidney transplants in the UK.

126 people received a pancreas or combined kidney/pancreas transplant–the highest number on record and an increase of 47% over the previous year.

586 patients received a liver transplant, 8% fewer than in the previous year.

262 cardiothoracic transplants were carried out, a decrease of 9% compared to the previous year, the decrease in heart and heart/lung transplants being marked.

At the end of March 2006, 6,700 patients were listed as actively waiting for a transplant, a 9% increase compared to the previous year.

A further 2,503 people had their sight restored through a cornea transplant–the highest number for 9 years.

Almost a million more people pledged to help others after their death by registering their wishes on the NHS Organ Donor Register

Note the increase in pancreas/kidney and the decrease of the heart/lung and liver transplantation.

Apart from the remarkable increase of kidney transplants from living donors, organ donation in the UK, as in most advanced countries, heavily depends on deceased heartbeating donors.

Table VII

TRANSPLANTATION FROM LIVING DONORS
(UK. 2005-2006)

Living Donors	2004-2005	2005-2006	% change
Kidney	475	579	22
Heart (**domino**)	1	0	-
Liver/Liver Lobe	7	9	-
Total Transplants	483	588	22

Table VIII

TRANSPLANTS FROM DECEASED DONORS
(UK. 2005-2006)

Deceased Donors	2004-2005	2005-2006	% change
Heartbeating	664	639	-4
Non-heartbeating	88	126	43
Total Donors	752	765	2

Tables VI, VII and VIII were reprinted by permission.
Statistics prepared by UK Transplant from the National Transplant Database maintained on behalf of transplant services in the UK and Republic of Ireland. UK statistics can be found at <http://www.uktransplant.org.uk/ukt/statistics/statistics. jsp>. UK Transplant is part of NHS Blood and Transplant (NHSBT).

The very important trend of organ transplantation has long passed the experimental stage and an increase in transplantation surgery will be characteristic of the future. Incurable diseases may become curable in many instances and useful life can be added to individuals who are suffering from end-stage diseases. One of the future concerns from the point of view of death and dying will be the ethical question of how much of a dead body can be used for transplantation without indignity. It is possible to foresee, in a futuristic way, that there will be fewer and fewer remains for burial and, maybe one day, almost the whole body will be used to help others to survive otherwise incurable diseases.

The concept of brain death and its practical consequences have become the *conditio sine qua non* of organ donation from deceased donors. This practice created not only a new science but also new hope for an ever increasing number of patients whose life could not be saved without using organ transplantation to replace a hopelessly diseased organ. The number of new trials is increasing every year and many of the recipients return to a healthy and active life after the replacement of a useless organ from the best source, the human deceased donors.

Transplantation of cadaver organs is legally permissible provided that it is done ethically. A prerequisite to the replacement of organs is to have the highest professional standards in tertiary care institutions, and equipment for the complex diagnostic and treatment modalities that are required for tissue typing and transplantation surgery. The paragraph that follows is from the World Medical Association's statement on human organ and tissue donation and transplantation, adopted by the 52nd WMA General Assembly in Edinburgh, Scotland during October 2000.[9]

Physicians have an obligation to ensure that interactions at the bedside, including those discussions related to organ donation, are sensitive and consistent with ethical principles and with their fiduciary obligations to their patients. This is particularly so given that conditions at the bedside of dying patients are not ideal for the process of free and informed decision making. Protocols should specify that whoever approaches the patient, family members or other designated decision makers about the donation of organs and tissues should possess the appropriate combination of knowledge, skill and sensitivity for engaging in such discussions. Medical students and practising physicians should seek the necessary training for this task, and the appropriate authorities should provide the resources necessary to secure that training.

The Canadian Medical Association's policy statement and Code of Ethics contains the following paragraphs that are highly relevant to this discussion:

CMA policy statement about transplantation

An ethical physician:

will allow death to occur with dignity and comfort when death of the body appears to be inevitable;

may, when death of the body has occurred, support cellular life in the body when some parts of the body might be used to prolong or improve the health of others;

will recognize his responsibility to a donor of organs to be transplanted and will give to the donor or his relatives full disclosure of his intent and the purpose of the procedure;

in the case of a living donor, he will also explain the risks of the procedure;

will refrain from determining the time of death of the donor patient when he will be participant in the performance of the transplant procedure or when his association with any proposed recipient might influence his judgement; who determined the time of death of the donor may, subsequent to the transplant procedure, treat the recipient.

CMA Code of ethics: (2006)

Responsibilities to the patient:

Communication, Decision Making and Consent

27. Ascertain wherever possible and recognize your patient's wishes about the initiation, continuation or cessation of life-sustaining treatment.

28. Respect the intentions of an incompetent patient as they were expressed (e.g. through a valid advance directive or proxy designation) before the patient became incompetent.

29. When the intentions of an incompetent patient are unknown and when no formal mechanism for making treatment decision is in place, render such treatment as you believe to be in accordance with the patient's values or, if these are unknown, the patient's best interest.

30. Be considerate of the patient's family and significant others and cooperate with them in the patient's interest.

Since organ transplantation from the deceased requires viable tissue—viability meaning that the organ was well perfused with oxygenated blood prior to removal from the body—it is important to discuss matters with the relatives in advance, explaining that the surgery to remove donated organs will take place after the patient has died. When death is certified, the attending physician should inform the relatives that their loved one is dead and this would be the last opportunity to see the body before it is taken for removal of the organs for transplantation. All questions should be answered with patience and compassion. Since the patient's wishes through advance directives (living will, power of attorney or discussion with the relatives) must have already been clarified, it would be unnecessary pressure to ask for their permission to turn off the respirator.

After the relatives have left the treatment area (usually the intensive care unit), artificial maintenance of circulation and oxygenation continues, sometimes for hours or until the surgery can be arranged. The implantation of the removed kidney or heart may take place in a neighboring operating room immediately or hours later, sometimes in another hospital or even another country. Removed organs can be perfused artificially and kept in sterile bags or sterile containers, packed in wet ice, placed in a cooler and transported to the transplant hospital. Viability can be maintained for several hours.

The limits of keeping brain-dead bodies on the respirator are unclear. Without using other supportive measures, cardiovascular collapse and cardiac arrest will occur within days. In exceptional cases (e.g. maternal brain death during pregnancy), much more time can be gained to facilitate survival of the foetus. Such cases are known from the medical literature (Dillon et al., 1982)[10] and (Field et al., 1988).[11]

Dillon's patient was a 24-year-old woman, admitted to hospital in **status epilepticus,** with the gestational age of the fetus at twenty-three weeks. Her seizures were well controlled with phenytoin until four months prior to the hospital admission. Initially, she had improved on the applied therapy, but on the fourteenth hospital day her condition deteriorated and required readmission to the ICU. By the seventeenth hospital day she was in unresponsive coma with fixed dilated pupils, intubated and on the respirator. On the nineteenth hospital day, after all required tests using brain-oriented criteria, she was pronounced dead. With continued assisted respiration, intravenous medication and hyperalimentation, life support of the fetus was maintained, but on the twenty-fourth hospital day the maternal blood pressure started to fall and because of fetal distress, a Caesarean section was performed at the bedside. The infant girl weighed 930 grams and in spite of numerous problems she was **extubated** at five weeks of age. Two months later she was discharged from the intensive care nursery, weighing approximately two kilograms.

Fields et al. published their case six years later. In this study, the patient was a 27-year-old primigravida (first pregnancy) at 22-week gestation who was admitted to hospital with a five-day history of severe headache, vomiting and disorientation. There were no focal neurological abnormalities. A lumbar puncture showed slightly elevated CSF pressure but no evidence of meningitis or subarachnoid hemorrhage. Four hours after admission, the patient had a generalized epileptic seizure and went into respiratory arrest. After a failed CPR she was declared brain-dead with continued life support for the fetus. After nine weeks, an apparently normal and healthy male infant weighing 1,440 grams was delivered by Caesarean section. Post-mortem examination showed **holonecrosis** of the mother's brain. The newborn did well and was growing and developing normally at 18 months of age. Although the technical aspects of prolonged life support demanded intensive care and the economic costs were very high ($217,784), there were ample ethical arguments to justify the separation of brain death and somatic death. The maintenance of the body of a brain-dead mother made it possible that her unborn fetus could develop and mature.

Transplant protocols are many; they represent ethical standards required by professional associations and many times by hospitals themselves. This field is still evolving with ongoing recommendations to standardize both the medical and surgical management of organ donation. A supplement of the *Canadian Medical Association Journal*[12] is a good example of a document which might lead to the formulation of a national practice standard in the field of ethical, professional and technical requirements of organ donation.

Notes

1. Byrne, P., Coimbra, C. G., Spaeman, R., Wilson, M. A., "Brain death" is not death! Essay at a meeting of the Pontifical Academy of Sciences, February, 2005. Dr. Paul Byrne, to Compassionate Healthcare Network, March 29, 2005 via e-mail. <http://chninternational.com/brain_death_is_not_death_byrne_paul_md.html>, accessed June 8, 2006.

2. Pope Pius XII, The Prolongation of Life: Allocution to the International Congress of Anesthesiologists, November 24, 1957, in *The Pope Speaks,* Vol. 4, (1958): 393-398.

3. Shemie, S. D., Doig, C., Dickens, B., et al., Severe brain injury to neurological determination of death: Canadian forum recommendations, *CMAJ,* 174(6), Suppl. (2006): S1-S12.
The full text of the document is accessible on the interenet: <http://www.cmaj.ca/cgi/content/full/174/6/S1>.

4. Capron, A. M., Brain Death: Well settled yet still unresolved (Editorial), *N Eng J Med,* 344, (2001): 1244-1246.

5. Shemie, S. D., Ross, H., Pagliarello, J., et al., Organ donor management in Canada: Recommendations of the forum on medical management to optimize donor organ potential, *CMAJ,* 174(6), (Suppl.), (2006): S13-S23.

6. Sheehy, E., Conrad, S. L., Brigham, L. E., et al., Estimating the number of potential organ donors in the United States, *N Engl J Med,* 349, (2003): 667-674.

7. Wood, K. E., Becker, B. N., McCartney, J. G., et al., Care of the potential organ donor, *N Engl J Med,* 351, (2004): 2730-2739.

8. Shemie, S. D., Doig, C., Belitsky, P., Advancing toward a modern death: the path from severe brain injury to neurological determination of death, *CMAJ,* 168(8), (2003): 993-995.

9. <http://wma.net/e/policy/wma.html>, accessed July 25, 2006.

10. Dillon, W. P., Lee, R. V., Tronolone, M. J., et al., Life support and maternal brain death during pregnancy, *JAMA*, 248, (1982): 1089-1091.

11. Field, D. R., Gates, E. A., Creasy, R. K., et al., Maternal brain death during pregnancy: Medical and ethical issues, *JAMA*, 260(6), (1988): 816-822.

12. See citation 5: Shemie, et al., *CMAJ*, 174(6), (Suppl.), (2006): S13-S23.

CHAPTER 5
THE VEGETATIVE STATE*

The persistent vegetative state (**PVS**), has been used as a clinical term to describe the unfortunate outcome that sometimes follows traumatic head injuries, or other acute insults to the brain (hemorrhage, anoxic/**ischemic** damage). It may also be the result of progressive, degenerative diseases (e.g. **Alzheimer's, Parkinson's** and others). The preferred diagnostic term today for the acute phase is vegetative state (**VS**), which may improve in time or may even progress to recovery with minor or major functional deficits. If the patient doesn't improve and remains in a vegetative state for a long period of time, the persistent or permanent modifier can be added to the descriptive term.

---

*When Jennett and Plum published their paper Persistent vegetative state after brain damage: a syndrome in search of a name, Lancet, 1, (1972): 734-737, they carefully explained that "vegetative itself is not obscure; vegetative is defined in the Oxford English Dictionary as 'to live a merely physical life, devoid of intellectual activity or social intercourse'. It suggests even to the layman a limited and primitive responsiveness to external stimuli; to the doctor it is also a reminder that there is relative preservation of autonomic regulation of the internal milieu."

Persistent vegetative state soon replaced all the previous terms (akinetic mutism, coma vigil, apallic syndrome) and became one of the most cited syndromes in the medical literature. It is unfortunate that the term "vegetative" which refers to the vegetative nervous system, and synonymous with the autonomic nervous system, acquired a pejorative overtone with the hidden meaning that the patient with this diagnosis is not a human being, not even an animal but a vegetable. Because of this concern Dossetor proposed the replacement of "vegetative state" with "incognitive state." (John B. Dossetor, CMA ETHICS Withdrawal of treatment: is it ever justifiable? Human Medicine, Volume 7 Number 1, 2007). It is regrettable that "incognitive state" has been used by philosophers with a different meaning and that the "vegetative state" is so deeply imbedded in the medical literature that it will probably be a long time before another, less offensive term will find its place in dictionaries.

How long should a person be in a vegetative state before we call it persistent remains a debatable point. An outstanding monograph on the subject, authored by Bryan Jennett,[1] discusses in a scholarly fashion "everything you ever wanted to know" about the condition. The vegetative state deserves close attention because it represents the conflict between respect for the sanctity of life and for the victim's autonomy and best interests, and between killing and letting die.

Definition

Although the condition has been known for over a century, a concise definition is hard to come by. The American Academy of Neurology (1989)[2] described PVS this way:

> The persistent vegetative state is a form of eyes-open permanent unconsciousness in which the patient has periods of wakefulness and physiological sleep/wake cycles, but at no time is the patient aware of him- or herself or the environment. Neurologically, being awake but unaware is the result of a functioning brainstem and the total loss of cerebral cortical functioning.

To draw the line between brain death and vegetative state, *Encyclopædia Britannica*[3] describes it as follows:

> [Patients] in persistent vegetative state: They breathe and swallow spontaneously, grimace in response to pain, and are clinically and electrophysiologically awake, but they show no behavioral evidence of awareness. Their eyes are episodically open (so that the term *coma* is inappropriate to describe them), but their retained capacity for consciousness is not endowed with any content. Some patients have remained like this for many years. Such patients are not dead, and their prognosis depends in large part on the quality of the care they receive. The discussion of their management occasionally abuts onto controversies about euthanasia and the "right to die". These issues are quite different from that of the "determination of

death", and failure to distinguish these matters has been the source of great confusion.

Historical evolution of the term and prevalence of the condition

In 1899, Rosenblath[4] had reported a 15-year-old patient with a very severe head injury who after two weeks in coma recovered, strangely awake, but died after eight months, though being tube fed in this state. In 1940 Kretschmer[5] described two patients suffering from severe brain damage who were awake, but not responding. He proposed the term "apallic syndrome" for the condition and this term was often used in Europe[6] in reference to the absent functions of the cerebral cortex, the outer layer of the brain, also known by the Latin *pallium cerebri* (the cerebral mantle).

In the United States, Cairns (1941)[7] coined the term "akinetic mutism", whereas in the French medical literature "coma vigil" was the preferred name. The term "Persistent Vegetative State" (PVS) was originally suggested by Jennett and Plum (1972)[8] to describe patients with irreversible brain damage, usually from trauma or hypoxic/ischemic insult to the brain. PVS and apallic syndrome (Ingvar et al.)[9] were interchangeable terms in the twentieth century, mostly in Europe. PVS may arise from three categorically different causes:

1. Chronic brain disorders, when the vegetative outcome is the final stage of a relentless downhill course; chronic conditions account for 25% of the cases. Among the chronic degenerative diseases that end in PVS, 50% originate in Alzeheimer's disease.
2. Acute, traumatic, and non-traumatic insults to the brain, when the vegetative outcome is the end result of recovery from deep coma. PVS arising from acute coma represents 75% of the cases (severe head injury 34.5% and non-traumatic coma 40%).
3. Congenital anomaly and birth trauma (**anencephaly** and neonatal asphyxia).

We have seen several dozen patients in vegetative state over a long neurosurgical practice. When the senior author first wrote about it (Ivan, 1990)[10] there were between 5,200 and 7,800 patients in a persistent vegetative state (PVS) in the United States and about 800 persons in Canada. The Multi-Society Task Force on the Persistent Vegetative State[11] estimated in 1994 that there were 10,000 to 25,000 adults and 4,000 to 10,000 children in persistent vegetative states in the United States.

The approximate expenditure for the yearly maintenance of vegetative lives, a condition quite rightly called "a fate worse than death",[12] was $40 to $80 million in Canada and about $1 billion in the United States.

The global prevalence of PVS is unknown.[13] This is because of the "lack of accepted diagnostic criteria and the fact that, until recently, neither the International Classification of Diseases (ICD-9-CM) nor most health agencies included persistent vegetative state as a codable diagnosis". The prevalence of PVS in Japan[14] is about 0.0025%, (2-3 per 100,000 population) which appears close to the estimates of other countries. At a casual glance this looks like a small figure but may represent a great financial burden for families or for the state. In a paper, "The six million dollar woman", Paris[15] describes a 27-year-old female patient who, after a head injury, lived in a vegetative state for 17 years, at an estimated cost of $6,104,590.

Neuropathology

Brain death and PVS are possible outcomes of the comatose states, but in brain death, the whole brain (both the cortex and the brainstem) are destroyed by a massive insult, anoxia, or injury, whereas in PVS the brainstem is spared. With brain death there is no spontaneous respiration; in PVS the brainstem maintains respiratory movements.

Since there are several possibilities (trauma, hemorrhage, inflammation, degenerative diseases and anoxia) that can cause the vegetative state, there are no clear and characteristic pathological pictures except for the obvious evidence of destruction of the cerebral cortex or its connections. The initial insult must have spared the lower brainstem which sustains functions that medical science calls vegetative, such as respiration and circulation, although in a few cases of PVS, incomplete damage to the brainstem was also reported at autopsy.

The anatomical basis for VS and PVS differs somewhat from case to case for several reasons. The interval between brain injury and death affects the nature and severity of pathologic changes. In patients with a chronic neurologic condition it may be difficult to determine at autopsy which neuropathologic changes were responsible for the initial failure to recover consciousness. Apart from the above limitations, two major patterns have characterized most reports both in post-traumatic and non-post-traumatic PVS. In the first, pathologists find changes in the grey matter (**diffuse laminar cortical necrosis**) following oxygen deprivation or failure of blood circulation (**global hypoxia** and ischemia), whereas in the second, after severe closed head injuries, disruption of the connecting fibres in the white matter (**diffuse axonal injury**) can be seen as a result of sheering forces that disrupted the connection between the grey matter (cortex) and the rest of the brain.

Diagnosis of the vegetative state

The accepted clinical parameters that define the vegetative state are: return of sleep/wake cycles, spontaneous maintenance of blood pressure and regular respiratory pattern, lack of discreet localizing motor responses, absence of vocalization, inability to obey commands, and lack of sustained visual pursuit movements. The patient is described as wakeful but devoid of conscious content and cognitive or affective functions.

The diagnosis is primarily clinical and requires a neurological examination and careful observation. The patient's face has a vacant look, the body is in a typical "**fetal posture**", the limbs are spastic, the spinal and brainstem reflexes are exaggerated, and there are usually purposeless chewing movements.

PVS must be distinguished from other prolonged states of lack of responsiveness; the most important of these is the "locked-in syndrome," in which part of the brainstem is damaged but the cortex is intact. Locked-in patients are able to communicate with a variety of signals usually indicating "yes" or "no" by blinking or making a left or right movement with their eyes. A striking example of this condition was Jean-Dominique Bauby, a French journalist and the editor of the magazine *Elle*, who at the age of 43 suffered a massive stroke. When he became conscious he could only move his head a little, grunt, and blink his left eyelid. Despite being in this locked-in condition, he authored the book *The Diving Bell and the Butterfly* by blinking when the correct letter was reached by a person reciting the alphabet.

The clinical course of vegetative states shows great variation. It can be transient in 1-14% of the patients following severe head trauma but, in the early few weeks of a post-traumatic coma, there are no good predictive criteria. Some evidence suggests that patients with decorticate posturing, respiratory dysfunction and other injuries to the body are more liable to go into vegetative state. Nevertheless, after a few weeks in a vegetative state some patients may recover. The probability of recovery becomes remote after a month and the patient would perhaps qualify for the diagnosis of persistent vegetative state. Even PVS patients have a small chance to improve, but after a year the vegetative state can justifiably be called permanent.

In case of doubt about the diagnosis and prognosis, certain investigative methods might be of some use. The CT scan is non-specific, although it may be helpful;[16] the EEG shows too many variations,[17] but the PET scan is quite specific. The cerebral metabolic rate for glucose is very low in PVS, whereas in the locked-in syndrome the cortical glucose metabolism is only slightly less than normal (Levy et al., 1987).[18]

The natural course of PVS

The prognosis and management of PVS is still debatable. Patients may survive almost indefinitely, so long as they receive adequate nutrition, a high standard of nursing care and protection against and treatment for infections. Nevertheless, even with good care, about 75% will have died at the end of five years.

The probability of improving, or regaining the cognitive state is very low. According to some important reports (Levy et al., 1978)[19] of those patients who were vegetative at one month, 87% were dead at one year; 5.5% remained vegetative and only two patients regained some awareness between one month and one year. Unexpected improvements occurred occasionally after many months, in one case after two years. None of these improvements resulted in independence.[20, 21, 22]

Is there a sure way to predict the possible vegetative outcome in an acute coma? Prediction of PVS with **somatosensory-evoked potentials** is highly accurate within eight hours after the onset of anoxic or cardiorespiratory coma both in children and adults. (Zegers et al.)[23], (Frank et al.)[24] Unfortunately, the same accuracy for outcome prediction is not true in coma of traumatic origin.

How accurately can we diagnose PVS and more importantly how persistent is PVS? The accuracy of the clinical diagnosis is extremely high, but the meaning of the term "persistent" is vague and debatable. The definition of persistent in *Webster's Third New International Dictionary* is, "continuing to exist in spite of interference or treatment". It is an excellent definition, but it does not specify any time element. After how many weeks, months, or years, can we call a condition persistent?

There is also a relatively new subgroup of patients with severe alteration of consciousness which may create disagreement among experts. These patients do not meet the diagnostic criteria for coma or vegetative state (Giacino et al., 2002)[25]. The condition is called the minimally conscious state (MCS) and it represents a borderline situation without established evidence-based guidelines for diagnosis.

These uncertainties demand extreme caution with the prognosis and management of patients in vegetative state.

With patients in acute coma, the first round of prognostication is an attempt to predict whether they will live, become vegetative, or die. In case of vegetative survival, we move into a second round of prognostication to predict persistence. At this stage of our knowledge, we can only say that if the vegetative state persists for three months, the probability is very high that it will either persist or the patient will die. However, even after one year, an occasional improvement can occur among those who remain vegetative.

So we have to live with probabilities and do what we can in the circumstances, because these patients are alive, although lacking quality in their existence. There are certain, albeit difficult ways, to consider them as potential organ donors. The Guidelines of the American Academy of Neurology[26] deal with the management of PVS including the criteria of withdrawing treatment.

The position paper of the Academy discusses the basic medical facts of PVS and explains why artificial nutrition and hydration are forms of medical treatment. It emphasizes the ethical position which supports the fundamental rights of patients to make their own decisions concerning treatment and attempts to reconcile the potential conflicts between the wishes and rights of the patients, their families, and the health care personnel.

The document reinforces the American Medical Association's position that:

1. Medical treatment includes artificial nutrition and hydration and,
2. Treatment may be stopped not only in patients who are terminally ill, but also in those who are in an irreversible coma.

According to these guidelines, if the patient is in a vegetative state, and his wishes are known, and the family requests discontinuation of treatment including hydration and nutrition, and the attending physician is in agreement, the patient may be allowed to die and thus may become a potential organ donor.

Apart from this eventuality, there is no other way to consider PVS patients as organ donors unless active euthanasia is legalized. Even then, further research has to determine the time when the vegetative state is considered irreversible with no chance of recovery. For practical purposes, we would suggest using the diagnosis of Vegetative State (VS) up to three months, Persistent Vegetative State (PVS) up to a year and **Permanent or Chronic Vegetative State (PerVS)** after one year without improvement.

If the senior author were asked by a young colleague how to relate to this difficult problem and how to handle PVS patients, he would give the following advice: (1) practice the American Academy of Neurology guidelines concerning the termination of useless treatment; (2) research further the predictive criteria of acute coma (particularly head injury); (3) explore the legalization and ethical acceptance of euthanasia as an act of ultimate kindness to terminate suffering and subhuman existence using the argument that society and the law should give PVS patients the right to die with dignity; and (4) keep PVS research independent from transplantation.

Well known cases of vegetative state

A review of the history of some well-known thoroughly scrutinized cases might give useful insight into the difficulties that relatives, health-care personnel and the courts have to face when they must try to choose the right action.

Karen Ann Quinlan was twenty-one years old when a tragic accident made her a central character in a conflict between the ability of modern medical technology to sustain life and her parents' wishes to allow a stricken daughter to die with peace and dignity.

In April 1975, Karen Ann had been partying with a small group of friends when, after accidentally ingesting a combination of prescription sedatives and alcohol, she had a cardiopulmonary arrest. She was found unresponsive, apnoeic, pulseless, and cyanotic with dilated pupils. Karen received cardiopulmonary resuscitation and was taken to the local hospital. In the emergency room, her pulse was present, but she was otherwise unchanged and was placed on a ventilator. On her second hospital day, because of aspiration pneumonia, a tracheostomy was performed and respiratory support continued.

Within several days she opened her eyes, but recovery of consciousness had not occurred and her physician came to the diagnosis that she was in a persistent vegetative state and informed her parents that their daughter had a "negligible chance of recovering to a cognitive, sapient state."[27]

Karen's parents were devout Catholics and had sought counsel with their parish priest before making any decision. Knowing what Karen would have wanted, that is, to remove her from the ventilator and let her die in peace, they were comforted to learn that church teaching supported their decision. Their position was based on a statement of Pope Pius XII when he addressed the conference of anesthesiologists in 1957. This is the relevant quotation of Pope Pius XII that applies to the Quinlans' request. *"The rights and the duties of the family depend in general upon the presumed will of the unconscious patient, if he is of age and 'sui juris'. Where the proper and independent duty of the family is concerned, they are usually bound only to the use of ordinary means."*[28]

After several months of waiting, the Quinlans asked the care givers to discontinue the use of the respirator, but the physicians and hospital administrators refused to honour their request. With the help of a lawyer, the Quinlans argued the case before a judge in the New Jersey Superior Court in October 1975. On October 10, the judge ruled against the Quinlans and the respiratory support had to continue.

The Quinlans appealed the decision and the case was argued before the seven judges of the New Jersey Supreme Court and by unanimous decision on January 17, 1976 they reversed the decision of the lower court. They also ruled that the ventilator could be removed only if Karen's physicians agreed that there was no likelihood of her recovery and that judgement was affirmed by an ethics committee.

The doctors refused to comply but the attending physician made attempts to wean her from the respirator. Several days of repeated attempts proved that she was able to breathe spontaneously and in a week's time she became respirator-independent.

In one year Karen's hospital expenses had reached $188,000 and since she was breathing on her own, transfer to a nursing home was arranged where she died in 1985, having never regained consciousness.

Her survival without a respirator was unexpected and so were the autopsy findings. As a detailed report in the New England Journal of Medicine informs us (Kinney et al., 1994)[29] the most severe changes were not in the cerebral cortex, but in the thalamus, a complex relay nucleus in the uppermost part of the brainstem. The lower brainstem with the respiratory centre was relatively intact.

The tragic case of this unfortunate young woman became a pivotal force to re-examine medical, legal and ethical problems that surround the diagnosis and management of the vegetative state. Hospitals developed Ethics Committees, Neurological Societies made practice guidelines and Medical Associations announced policy statements about ordinary and extraordinary measures in health care and end-of-life decisions in general. As often happens, guidelines bring forth dissenting voices and disagreements about life and suffering and, as of 2006, the sanctity of life versus the quality of existence still continues.

The next publicly discussed case was even more controversial in some respects.

Nancy Cruzan was a married woman, 25 years old, when in January 1983 she lost control of her car and landed face down in a water-filled ditch. When paramedics found her she had no detectable vital signs, but after resuscitation, her breathing and heartbeat returned while still at the accident site. She was transported to a hospital where a neurosurgeon diagnosed her as having sustained cerebral contusion compounded by significant cerebral anoxia. Her deep coma showed only minimal improvement and nine months after the accident, she was still in persistent vegetative state. Surgeons inserted a feeding tube for long-term care but efforts of rehabilitation failed and after four years her husband and her parents accepted that there was no hope for recovery. They requested removal of the feeding tube, but the hospital demanded a court order to that effect.

The Cruzan family's pursuit of a court order to have the feeding tube removed turned into a three-year, widely publicized struggle. On the basis of a friend's testimony that Nancy would not have wished to continue her life on artificial support, the trial court allowed the removal of the feeding tube. The Missouri State Supreme court reversed this decision ruling that the lower court did not meet the *clear and convincing evidence* standard. The U.S. Supreme Court affirmed the Missouri Supreme Court's ruling.[30]

The opinion of the U.S. Supreme Court stated:

". . . for purposes of this case, we assume that the United States Constitution would grant a competent person a constitutionally protected right to refuse lifesaving hydration and nutrition."

The Court noted that ". . . most state courts have based a right to refuse treatment on the common law right to informed consent . . . or on both that right and a constitutional privacy right."

But the Court also held that Missouri was correct to require a standard of:

". . . clear and convincing evidence" and that "the State may properly decline to make judgments about the 'quality' of a particular individual's life and simply assert an unqualified interest in the preservation of human life to be weighed against the constitutionally protected interests of the individual."

The three dissenting Justices argued on this basis:

"Medical technology has effectively created a twilight zone of suspended animation where death commences while life, in some form, continues. Some patients however, want no part of a life sustained only by medical technology. Instead, they prefer a plan of medical treatment that allows nature to take its course and permits them to die with dignity."

It maybe is enlightening to quote from Blackmun, one of

the dissenting justices, who, among other arguments, stated as follows:

"The Cruzan family appropriately came before the court seeking relief. The circuit judge properly found the facts and applied the law. His factual findings are supported by the record and his legal conclusions by overwhelming weight of authority. The principal opinion attempts to establish absolutes, but does so at the expense of human factors. In so doing it unnecessarily subjects Nancy and those close to her to continuous torture which no family should be forced to endure."

After the US Supreme Court's ruling, three close friends of Nancy Cruzan came forward with evidence that her wishes expressed when she was competent were that she would want the tube removed. The lower court then ruled this was clear and convincing evidence, and the decision was not appealed. Nancy Cruzan's feeding tube was taken out in December 1990. Fifteen members of "Operation Rescue", appeared at the hospital to re-insert the feeding tube, but they were arrested. Nancy died 11 days later on December 26, 1990.

As suggested by Fulton and Metress, whose several page analysis detailed the history of the Cruzan family's ordeal "The major lesson to be learned from the Cruzan case is quite simple; write it down." (Fulton, 1995).[31] In other words, a Living Will or Advance Directive might help to avoid court interference with the dignity of dying and block the intrusion of the media into the privacy of the bereaved family.

Terri Schiavo was born as Theresa Marie Schindler on December 3, 1963, to prosperous and devout Catholic parents.[32] She was a normal healthy child, but in her teens she had gained more weight than she wanted. The summer she graduated from high school, she went on a diet and began to lose weight. In the fall of the same year, she enrolled in the two-year program at Bucks County Community College, where, in a psychology class during her second semester, she met Michael Schiavo. They married two years later in 1984, when she was just under 21, eight months younger than Michael.

The young couple lived with Terri's parents in a Philadelphia suburb and two years later they all moved to St Petersburg,

Florida, where February 25, 1990 marked the onset of their ordeal. Terri was 27 years old when she had a cardiac arrest, triggered by extreme hypokalemia (potassium imbalance) brought on by an eating disorder and related to her diet (Quill, 2005).[33] As a result, severe hypoxic-ischemic encephalopathy developed, and during the subsequent months she exhibited no evidence of higher cortical function.

Computed tomographic (CT) scans of her brain showed severe atrophy of her cerebral hemispheres and her electroencephalograms (EEG) were flat, indicating no functional activity of the cerebral cortex. Her neurologic examinations were indicative of a persistent vegetative state. Those who were not familiar with the condition must have been impressed by the video clips so often shown on various TV channels as proof of her responsiveness. But two neurologists, selected by Michael Schiavo and one by the court agreed that the condition met the criteria of persistent vegetative state. The radiologist and the neurologist chosen by Terri's parents and siblings disagreed and suggested that her condition might improve with certain, unproven, therapies.

In May 1998, Michael Schiavo filed a petition in court to determine whether Terri's feeding tube should be removed. He took the position that Terri would choose to have the tube removed. The parents took the position that Terri would choose not to have the tube removed.

Following the trial, Judge Greer ruled that "clear and convincing evidence" showed that Terri would choose not to receive life prolongation medical care under her current circumstances (i.e., that she would choose to have the tube removed.).[34] Terri's feeding tube was removed for the first time on April 24, 2001. The Schindlers filed a civil suit against Michael alleging perjury, which was assigned to another court. The judge, Frank Quesada, issued an injunction against removal of the feeding tube until this was settled. The feeding tube was reinserted on April 26.

The relationship between Michael Schiavo and the Schindlers began breaking down earlier, in 1993. Mr Schiavo attempted to refuse treatment when his wife had an infection. The Schindlers took legal action to order treatment and this became the beginning of a wide-ranging, acrimonious series of legal and public opinion battles that eventually involved multiple special-interest groups. It was not only the media, but religious, ethical and medical groups with their forums and journals that became participants in an unending battle with a variety of opposing views. Michael Schiavo was criticized for being motivated by financial greed. His loyalty was questioned because he lived with another woman. The Schindlers received criticism for not accepting Terri's irremediable condition and fighting for their own wishes and values rather than yielding to hers.

After numerous injunctions and challenges of the rulings the feeding tube was removed for the second time in October 2003. This was followed, by the creation of "Terri's Law" by the Florida Legislature to permit the Governor to issue a stay in cases like Terri's and restore her feeding tube. The Governor signed the bill into law and immediately ordered a stay. Terri was moved from the nursing home and briefly hospitalized while her feeding tube was restored for the second time. From December 2003 to March 31, 2005 one lawsuit followed another when, with extreme media attention, human dignity and the right to privacy vanished and the tragedy of the life of an unfortunate dying young woman was turned into a spectator sport.

Finally, on March 18, 2005, Terri's feeding tube was removed for the third time but the fight continued daily between the Schindlers and various courts until the Supreme Court's final decision to deny the reinsertion of the feeding tube. The next day, March 31, 2005, Terri Schiavo passed away.

Can patients, doctors, politicians, orthodox thinkers and extremists learn anything from the life and death of Terri Schiavo? The answer is easier for patients and doctors. For patients and the public at large, the best advice is "write down your wishes". Be it a simple statement on a paper, a living will or an advance directive made by a lawyer, it could make a difference. All of these documents help the doctors, the family—and if it comes to it—the courts, to support a patient's wishes. The doctor has the obligation to respect the law and the ethical norms of the medical profession that do not allow treatment against the will of a patient or his/her guardian.

For the ethicists, religious leaders and zealous activists, the case of Terri Schiavo became a barricade to reinforce and defend. Instead of trying to play the role of arbiters, we will simply present the following range of quotes to show the complexity of the issues.

In an article that appeared in the *New England Journal of Medicine* under the heading of "Legal Issues in Medicine" the author (Annas, 2005)[35] states:

> Most Americans will agree with a resolution that was overwhelmingly adopted by the California Medical Association on the same day that Congress passed the Schiavo law: *Resolved: That the California Medical Association expresses its outrage at Congress' interference with these medical decisions.*

A Gallup poll (Moore, 2005)[36] conducted in May 2005 asked the following hypothetical question:

> If you personally were in a persistent vegetative state with no hope for significant recovery, would you want to have your life support removed, or not? 84.91% said yes, 13.06% said no.

Focusing on Terri Schiavo the question was:

> As you may know, the feeding tube that was keeping Terri Schiavo alive was removed. Based on what you have heard or read about the case, do you think that the feeding tube should or should not have been removed? 56% of Americans agreed that it was the right thing to do, while 31% disagreed.

In the *British Medical Journal*, under "News" one author states:

> While the wrangling in Washington continued, President Bush said, "The case of Terri Schiavo raises complex issues. Yet in instances like this one, where there are serious questions and substantial doubts, our society, our laws, and our courts should have a presumption in favor of life." Arthur Caplan, director of the Center for Bioethics at University of Pennsylvania, said the Schiavo case had already received ample scrutiny. Over the years it had come before nineteen judges and six courts. "It has been the most extensively litigated right-to-die case in the history of the United States." (Charatan, 2005)[37]

The following statement appeared in an editorial in the *Canadian Medical Association Journal*: "The sacred and the secular: the life and death of Terri Schiavo" (CMAJ, 2005).[38]

One paragraph states:

> Despite multiple appeals to the courts, the Schiavo case has created no major legal precedence in the US, but Schiavo's very public death may well set in motion legislative changes to satisfy those who would like to translate all knotty questions into the rhetoric of a culture of life.

And further in the editorial the writer makes this judgement:

> Few of us could honestly say that we would prefer governments and courts never to weigh in on questions concerning the sanctity and dignity of life, never to exert a protective influence in these matters. But there seems little doubt that, in North America, ideology and religion have begun to seriously distort the type of consensus-building that is the proper business of democratic politics.

The postmortem examination of Terri Schiavo was discussed in a Hastings Center Report (Fins and Schiff, 2005).[39]

> The autopsy reported that at her death, Terri Schiavo had a brain weight of 615 grams, half that of a normal brain and significantly less than Karen Ann Quinlan's, which weighed 835 grams. She had developed hydrocephalus *ex vacuo*, a condition marked by enlarged ventricles filled with **cerebrospinal fluid**, because of the profound loss of cortical volume.

And further, the authors comment:

> Remarkably, her brain showed a total loss of basal ganglia neurons, and her thalamus was "similarly affected".
> These observations are consistent with Jennett's research on the pathology of the vegetative state. He has noted that in nontraumatic cases of PVS, "the damage is usually extensive necrosis in the cerebral cortex, almost always associated with thalamic damage".

The statement of Pope John Paul II is available from various sources. We cite here part of the Illinois Right to Life Committee's webpage:[40]

> Pope John Paul II stated that removal of feeding tubes from people in vegetative states is immoral, and that no judgment on their quality of life could justify such "euthanasia by omission". John Paul made the comments to participants at a March 20, 2004 Vatican conference on the ethical dilemmas of dealing with incapacitated patients. The Pope said even the medical terminology used to describe people in so-called "persistent vegetative states" was degrading to them. He said no matter how sick a person was, "he is and will always be a man, never becoming a 'vegetable' or 'animal'".

William E. May, Professor of Moral Theology at the Catholic University of America, published *Human Existence and Ethics: Reflections on Human Life* in 1977. In the book he commented on the Karen Quinlan case, stating that there was no obligation "to use the means currently employed to prolong her death". He claimed that it would be morally permissible for her parents and others to "remove the tubes necessary for her feeding, prevent hydration by appropriate medical means, and attend to her dying moments."

In 1985 the Pontifical Academy of Sciences released a report on the artificial prolongation of life with the declaration that "if the patient is in a permanent, irreversible coma, as far as can be foreseen, treatment is not required, but all care should be lavished on him, including feeding." (May, 2005)[41] This prompted Professor May to reconsider the position he had taken in 1977. This long document, of 25 pages, explains why he and Germain Grisez changed their views in favour of continuing the tube feeding. Two dissenting Dominicans, Benedict Ashley and Kevin O'Rourke, did not change their stand and maintained that food and nutrition constituted extraordinary care and could be morally omitted.

So, it appears that the issue of ordinary and extraordinary means requires further elucidation and understanding. Opinion polls tell us that the vast majority of people would not like to continue living in a vegetative state. The courts base their decisions on clear and convincing evidence that the unconscious patient would choose a course of being allowed to die if living means only in vegetative state. Even high-ranking Catholic clergy vacillate between the statements of Pope Pius XII and Pope John Paul II.

We have already alluded to one of the main arguments that remains of O'Rourke. Pius XII had this to say:

> . . . normally one is held to use only ordinary means [to prolong life]–according to the circumstances of persons, places, times, and culture–that is to say, means that do not involve any grave burdens for oneself or another. A more strict obligation would be too burdensome for most men and would render the attainment of the higher, more important good too difficult. Life, health, all temporal activities are in fact subordinated to spiritual ends. On the other hand, one is not forbidden to take more than the strictly necessary steps to preserve life and health so long as he does not fail in some more important duty.

Pope John Paul's statement came at the conclusion of an international congress on March 20, 2004. Among other statements he said:[42]

> I should like to underline how the administration of food and water, even when provided by artificial means, always represents a natural means of preserving life, not a medical act. Its use, furthermore, should be considered, in principle, ordinary and proportionate, and as such, morally obligatory, insofar as and until it is seen to have attained its proper finality, which in the present case consists in providing nourishment to the patient and alleviation of suffering.

Thus it remains an unresolved issue, whether the withdrawal of food and fluid in the vegetative state is an act of ultimate kindness arising from the love and respect for the dying person or whether it is an immoral act as judged by those who believe that the quality of human existence cannot prevail over the sanctity of life.

To describe the presently prevailing contradicting views it might be appropriate here to quote the first sentence from a book authored by an expert, who has seen and written more than most of us about the vegetative state (Jennett, 2002).[43]

The strange and harrowing sight of a person being awake but unaware with no evidence of a working mind–characteristics of the vegetative state–provokes intense debate and raises profound questions for health professionals, ethicists, philosophers and lawyers.

And, if we may add, when there is a conflict between these views and their resolution reaches the courts, the decision of the judges is often more debatable. In most countries where doctor-assisted suicide is a criminal offence, withholding fluid from an incognitive patient becomes an act of kindness and tolerated by the law.

Notes

1. Jennett, B., *The Vegetative State: Medical facts, ethical and legal dilemmas* (Cambridge: Cambridge University Press, 2002).

2. Position of the American Academy of Neurology on certain aspects of the care and management of the persistent vegetative state patient. Adopted by the Executive Board, American Academy of Neurology, April 21, 1988, Cincinnati, OH, *Neurology*, 39, (1989): 125-126.

3. death, in *Encyclopædia Britannica* <http://www.britannica.com/eb/article-22180>, accessed June 13, 2006.

4. Rosenblath, W., Über einen bermerkenswerten Fall von Hirnerschütterung, *Dtsch Arch Klin Med*, 64, (1899): 406-429.

5. Kretschmer, E., Das apallische Sydrom, *Zbl Gesamte Neurol Psychiatr Berlin*, 169, (1940): 576-579.

6. Ore, G. D., Gerstenbrand, F., Lucking, C. H., *The Apallic Syndrome* (Berlin: Springer-Verlag, 1977).

7. Cairns, H., Oldenfield, R. C., Pennybacker, J. B., et al., Akinetic mutism with an epidermoid cyst of the third ventricle, *Brain*, 64, (1941): 273-290.

8. Jennett, B., Plum, F., Persistent vegetative state after brain damage: A syndrome in search of a name, *Lancet*, 1, (1972): 734-737.

9. Ingvar, D. H., Brun, A., Johansson, L., Samuelsson, S. M., Survival after severe cerebral anoxia with destruction of the cerebral cortex: the apallic syndrome, *Ann NY Acad Sci*, 315, (1978): 184-214.

10. Ivan, L. P., The persistent vegetative state, *Transplant Proc, 22,* (1990): 993-994.

11. The Multi-Society Task Force on PVS. Medical aspects of the persistent vegetative state, *New Engl J Med,* 330, (1994): 1499-1508.

12. Feinberg, W. M., Ferry, P. C., A fate worse than death. The persistent vegetative state in childhood, *Am J Dis Child,* 38(2), (1984): 128-130.

13. The Multi-Society Task Force on PVS. Medical aspects of the persistent vegetative state. *New Engl J Med,* 330, (1994): 1503.

14. Higashi, K., Hatano, M., Abiko, S., et al., Five year follow-up study of the patients with persistent vegetative state, *J Neurol Neurosurg and Psychiatry,* 44, (1981): 552-554.

15. Paris J. J., The six million dollar woman, *Conn Med,* 45, (1981): 720-721.

16. Young, R. S., Phelan, K. W., Lehman, R. A., et al., Computed tomographic findings in akinetic mutism, *Am J Dis Child,* 138, (1984): 166-167.

17. Hansotia, P. L., Persistent vegetative state. Review and report of electrodiagnostic studies in eight cases, *Arch Neurol,* 42, (1985): 1048-1052.

18. Levy, D. E., Sidtis, J. J., Rottenberg, D. A., et al., Differences in cerebral blood flow and glucose utilization in vegetative versus locked-in patients, *Ann Neurol,* 22, (1987): 673-682.

19. Levy, D. E., Knill-Jones, R. P., Plum, F., The vegetative state and its prognosis following nontraumatic coma, *Ann NY Acad Sci,* 315, (1978): 293-306.

20. Arts, W. F. M., Van Dongen, H. R., et al., Unexpected improvement after prolonged post traumatic vegetative state, *J Neurol Neurosurg and Psychiatry,* 48, (1985): 1300-1303.

21. Rosenberg, G. A., Johnson, S. F., Brenner, R. P., Recovery of cognition after prolonged vegetative state, *Ann Neurol,* 2, (1977): 167-168.

22. Shuttleworth, E., Recovery to social and economic independence from prolonged postanoxic vegetative state, *Neurology,* 33, (1983): 372-374.

23. Zegers de Beyl, D., Brunko, E., Prediction of chronic vegetative state with somatosensory evoked potentials, *Neurology,* 36, (1986): 134.

24. Frank, L. M., Furgiuele, T. L., Etheridge, Jr., J. E., Prediction of chronic vegetative state in children using evoked potentials, *Neurology,* 35, (1985): 931-934.

25. Giacino, J. T., Ashwal, S., Childs, N. et al., The minimally conscious state: Definition and diagnostic criteria, *Neurology,* 58, (2002): 349-353.

26. See note 2.

27. Fulton, G. B., Metress, E. K., *Perspectives on Death and Dying* (Boston: Jones and Bartlett, 1995): 72-75. This outstanding book gives a detailed description of several cases of vegetative states including Karen Ann Quinlan's.

28. Pope Pius XII, The Prolongation of Life: Allocution to the International Congress of Anesthesiologists, November 24, 1957, in *The Pope Speaks*, Vol. 4, (1958): 397.

29. Kinney, H. C., Korein, J., Panigrahy, A., et al., Neuropathological findings in the brain of Karen Ann Quinlan: The role of the thalamus in persistent vegetative state, *N Engl J Med*, 330, (1994): 1470-75.

30. Cruzan, by her parents and co-guardians v. Director, Missouri Department of Health, 497 U.S. 261, June 25, 1990, (Supreme Court of the United States).

31. Fulton, G. B., Metress, E. K., *Perspectives on Death and Dying* (Boston: Jones and Bartlett, 1995): 84-91.

32. Didion, J., The case of Theresa Schiavo, *The New York Review of Books*, LII, No. 10, (June 9, 2005).

33. Quill, T. E., Terri Schiavo: A tragedy compounded, *N Engl J Med*, 352, (2005): 1630-1633.
Dr. Quill is a professor of medicine, psychiatry, and medical humanities and the director of the Centre for Palliative Care and Clinical Ethics at the University of Rochester Medical Center, Rochester, NY.

34. Conigliaro, M., Abstract Appeal, Schiavo <http://abstractappeal.com/schiavo/infopage.html>, accessed June 21, 2006.

35. Annas, G. J., "Culture of Life" Politics at the Bedside: The Case of Terri Schiavo, *N Engl J Med*, 352, (2005): 1710-1715.

36. Moore, D. W., Public supports removal of feeding tube for Terri Schiavo, *Gallup News Service*, (March 22, 2005) <http://poll.gallup.com/content/default.aspx?ci=15310&pg=1&VERSION=p>, accessed June 23, 2006.

37. Charatan, F., President Bush and Congress intervene in "right to die" case, *BMJ*, 330, (2005): 687.

38. Editorial. The sacred and the secular: The life and death of Terri Schiavo, *CMAJ*, 172(9), (2005): 1149.

39. Fins , J. J., Schiff, N. D., In brief: The afterlife of Terri Schiavo, *The Hastings Center Report*, (2005) <http://www.medscape.com/viewarticles/511647> accessed June 24, 2006.

40. Pope Paul II declares feeding tube removal immoral. Right to Life Committee

Spring/Summer 2004. IRLC News <http://www.illinoisrighttolife.org/2004_2Fee
dingTubeRemovalImmoral.html>, accessed June 24, 2006.

41. May, W. E., Caring for persons in the "persistent vegetative state" and Pope
John Paul II's March 20, 2004 address "On life sustaining treatments and the
vegetative state", (October 23, 2005) <http://www.christendom-awake.org/pages/
may/caringforpersons.html>, accessed June 24, 2006.

42. Ibid.

43. Jennett, B., *The Vegetative State: Medical facts, ethical and legal dilemmas*
(Cambridge: Cambridge University Press, 2002).

CHAPTER 6
EUTHANASIA

None of the end-of-life dilemmas have polarized public opinion, ethical concerns and the law more than the question of euthanasia. It has been difficult to navigate through the hundreds of articles and dozens of books without losing faith that the conflicting ideas which surround assisted suicide may one day be resolved. When confronted by powerful arguments in favour of or against helping somebody die, one learns, with humility, that honesty and deep convictions motivate most of the opposing views. This chapter guides you through the maze of historical facts, legal arguments and ethical problems that lie at the core of the raging public debates.

Definition

The word euthanasia from Greek, simply means "pleasant death."

Webster's Third New International Dictionary defines euthanasia as

1: an easy death or means of inducing one; 2: the act or practice of painlessly putting to death persons suffering from incurable conditions or diseases.

The American Heritage Dictionary states[1]

The act or practice of ending the life of an individual suffering from a terminal illness or an incurable condition, as by lethal injection or the suspension of extraordinary medical treatment.

The definitions have various overtones, interpretations and connotations. They are: 1. making death less painful, 2. letting die, 3. actively helping to die, 4. mercy killing, and even the discredited view of 5. eugenics.

Making death less painful

Making death less painful or "agathanasia" (a term suggested by Paul Ramsey, a Protestant moral philosopher) is a practice which is characteristically used in palliative care units and hospices, where dying patients are treated symptomatically. This frequently involves the generous but judicious use of analgesic medications in conjunction with physical and spiritual support.

Letting die

Passive euthanasia, or "letting die" is a much more accepted way of responding to suffering. This means that certain treatments, sometimes classified as extraordinary means among the circumstances, are omitted. For example, the administration of antibiotics for pneumonia or the treatment of certain other complications of those suffering from a terminal illness may be withheld to avoid prolonging the dying process.

Actively helping to die

Active euthanasia is aimed directly at achieving the end of life. It usually occurs with the cooperation of health professionals who administer a lethal or excessive dose of a medication, such as barbiturates or morphine, to a dying patient or to a severely disabled person whose life is judged miserable or who request an end to their suffering. This act is homicide and, apart from a few countries in Europe, neither the law nor medical ethics are tolerant of this mercy.[2]

Mercy killing

Mercy killing is an act of compassionate murder usually committed by a close relative who decides abruptly to terminate the incurable state and the long suffering of a loved one, partner, sibling, or child by shooting, drowning, poisoning or some other method. The act is never concealed and the relative usually reports him or herself to the police. The charge is either murder or manslaughter, but because of the extenuating circumstances the minimal sentence prescribed by law for the crime would be applied in most cases.

Eugenics

Francis Galton coined the term "eugenics" in 1883, referring to efforts to improve the biological quality of future generations (Dowbiggin, 2005).[3] The negative connotations of the term come from Hitler's secret order which allowed Nazi doctors to "euthanize" mentally and physically handicapped patients. The revulsion stemming from this historical fact remains one of the most powerful and emotional arguments against euthanasia.

The roots and growth of the pro-euthanasia movement

We have reconstructed a short chronology of some landmarks in the history of euthanasia from the *Encyclopædia Britannica*,[4] Medina,[5] Humphry,[6] and Dowbiggin[7] as follows:

> The opinion that euthanasia is morally permissible is traceable to Socrates, Plato, and the Stoics.

> Suetonius, a Roman Historian (second century A.D) was the first to use the word euthanasia (Erdemir and Elcioglu)[8].

> After Suetonius, the philosopher Francis Bacon (1571-1626)

was the next in history to use the term "euthanasia". He advocated an *easy death* by mitigating pain.

The 18th century marked the first voices in favour of a humane way of dying. In his *Oratio de Euthanasia* (1794) the physician Paradys recommends easy death for those who are incurably ill or suffering.

To Voltaire (1694-1778), Montesquieu (1689-1755) and others of the Enlightenment, suicide was chiefly a matter of individual liberty.[9] The Scottish philosopher David Hume (1711-1776), defended suicide more strongly than Voltaire, but because of his reluctance to face opposition, his *Essays on Suicide* were published posthumously.

In 1931 C. Killick Millard (1870-1952), physician and researcher, drafted a bill attempting to legalize voluntary euthanasia in the UK and in 1935 founded the Voluntary Euthanasia Legalization Society (VELS).

The Societies bill was defeated in the House of Lords in 1936, as was a motion on the same subject in the House of Lords in 1950.

In the United States the Euthanasia Society of America was founded in 1938.

In 1997 Oregon became the first state in the United States to decriminalize physician-assisted suicide. Opponents of the controversial law, however, attempted to have it overturned.

The first countries to legalize euthanasia were the Netherlands on April 1, 2002 and Belgium on May 16, 2002.

In 1938 the Euthanasia Society of America (ESA) came into existence through the efforts of Ann Mitchell, a wealthy New Yorker and Charles Potter, the Unitarian minister, who in 1929, founded the First Humanist Society of New York. The Humanist Manifesto, scripted by two Unitarian ministers, C. W. Reese and J. H. Dietrich, was signed by the founder, Potter and sixty Unitarian pastors in 1933. Other members of the society included John Dewey, Albert Einstein, Julian Huxley and Thomas Mann. By 1937 the membership of the

Humanist Society in England, France, Australia and Russia had grown to about 15,000.

Exit International is a pro euthanasia organization founded in 1996 by Dr Philip Nitschke, the first doctor to give legal voluntary euthanasia under the Rights of the Terminally Ill Act of the Northern Territory in Australia. Based in Darwin, Exit International which now operates globally, was previously known as Exit Australia and the Voluntary Euthanasia Research Foundation.[10]

The ethical roots of anti-euthanasia

"Thou shalt not kill" (Exodus 20:13) is the most commonly quoted commandment from the Old Testament when debating justified or unjustified types of killing. Both Judaism and Islam teach that human life is sacred and they forbid suicide and euthanasia under any circumstances. Most Christian denominations adopted the tenet of the "sanctity of life" and some churches denied a Christian burial for those who had committed suicide. In many countries suicide became a criminal act.

Hippocrates, the Greek physician and the Father of Medicine (460-377 B.C.), established a medical school in Cos that forbade doctors to aid suicide. Aristotle (384-322 B.C.), the Greek philosopher and the author of *Ethics,* condemned suicide.

The famous French surgeon Ambroise Paré (1517-1590), one of the pioneers of the Renaissance, stated "Every individual has the right to live; only God creates human beings and death is the wish of God."

Catholic opposition to intentional killing is well supported in several papers and books. In Catholic teaching life is seen not as "self-creation" but as a gift of the Creator, a gift over which we are to exercise stewardship, not dominion (Paris and Moreland,

2005).[11] The authors point out that "supporters of assisted suicide overemphasize personal autonomy and wrongly delegate end-of-life decisions to physicians, thus violating the sovereignty of God over life". Further, they explain that the distinction made by the courts between withdrawal of medical support, which the Catholic Church sanctions, and actively aiding suicide, which it rejects, is central to Catholic theology.

Not all the arguments against euthanasia are religiously motivated. Secular ethicists have their say too in opposition to euthanasia and suicide. One such argument was made almost 50 years ago (Kamisar, 1958).[12] He suggested that the major arguments against euthanasia are:

- the likely high incidence of mistakes: medical error in diagnosis, irrational choices by those in pain or stress,
- the slippery slope of what is voluntary today could become involuntary tomorrow.

Medical doctors joined the anti-euthanasia movement in the First Do No Harm organization.[13] The organization, still functioning, was an offshoot of the World Federation of Doctors Who Respect Human Life, which

> [was] founded by Dutch doctors who had experience of the necessity to dissent from the Nazi Physicians Bureau and its social hygiene measures, and saw that traditional service to life was again endangered. Social policies of population control being planned by the U.N. World Population Conference in Bucharest in 1974 would include abortion, euthanasia and eugenics. A submission was made to the Conference on behalf of 70,000 doctors.

The enrolment form for the organization states:

> I support the World Medical Association's Declaration of Geneva, 1948. I am opposed to any action or omission which is intended to cause the death of a person. No one should be deprived of legal protection on grounds of age or disability.

The organization strongly opposes the British Medical Association's 1999 Guidelines which approved the withholding of fluids from victims of a stroke[14] and similar advice by the General Medical Council in 2002.[15]

On June 30, 2006 the *Chicago Tribune* reported that at the annual conference of the BMA, which represents about 135,000 doctors across the United Kingdom, about 65% of delegates voted to overturn the group's year-old policy of being neutral on the question of legalizing euthanasia. British doctors voted to restore their long-standing policy of opposing euthanasia.[16] At the same time, advocates of medically-assisted suicide accused religious groups of exerting undue influence over the vote.

A large number of doctors and nurses have written papers in various journals, both opposing and supporting euthanasia. The correspondence between two physicians in the *Canadian Medical Association Journal* (Lovrics[17] and Gorman,[18] 1999) provides an example of two opposing stands. Dr. Lovrics is a surgeon and an intensive care physician with considerable experience of withholding or withdrawing treatment. His letter is a comment on Daniel Gorman's essay on active and passive euthanasia. In support of palliative care Lovrics wrote:

> [Palliative care] does not relinquish the duty of care, rather, changes it to provide a peaceful, pain-free death . . . This is in stark contrast to euthanasia, which is a deliberate act to end life . . . The distinction between good palliative care and euthanasia (active or passive) or physician-assisted suicide is clear and important, not just semantics.

Two months later the CMA Journal published Gorman's reply in which he repeated his assertion that:

> . . . virtually everyone already supports passive euthanasia–regardless of what they prefer to call it–and that, in certain circumstances, the distinction between passive and active euthanasia is morally irrelevant. When our efforts to relieve suffering with palliative care fail, active euthanasia may be morally permissible and even preferred over passive euthanasia, for it ends suffering more quickly. . . . When we cannot, despite

our best efforts, adequately control the suffering of terminally
ill patients who want to die, active euthanasia may be a means
to respect their autonomy and relieve their distress.

Since so many contentious issues about end-of-life decisions
have been settled in the courts, we should examine the legal status of
euthanasia in a number of countries.

Euthanasia and the law

Canada

The Law Reform Commission (1983)[19] addressed euthanasia
with the following conclusions:

> *The voluntary aspect:* "The Commission recommends against
> legalizing or decriminalizing voluntary active euthanasia in any
> form and is in favour of continuing to treat it as a culpable
> homicide."

> *The mercy aspect:* "The Commission recommends that mercy
> killing not be made an offence separate from homicide and that
> there be no formal provision for special modes of sentencing
> for this type of homicide other than what is already provided
> for homicide."

> *Aiding suicide:* "The Commission . . . recommends retaining
> section 224 of the Criminal Code. It therefore recommended
> that the existing prohibitions in the Criminal Code concerning
> homicide be maintained."

Considering the problem of cessation of treatment (letting die), the
Commission stated:

> the decision to terminate, or not initiate useless treatment is
> sound medical practice and should be legally recognized as

such. The law, then, should not begin from the principle that a doctor who fails to prolong life acts illegally but rather, from the principle that a doctor acts legally if he does not prolong death.

Canada decriminalized suicide and attempted suicide in 1972, but assisted suicide and mercy killing are criminal offences.

In the early 1990s, 42-year-old Sue Rodriguez, who had amyotrophic lateral sclerosis (ALS or Lou Gehrig's disease), fought to overturn the law against assisted suicide. She lost her court battle, but was assisted in her dying with the help of an anonymous doctor. Under Canada's Criminal Code, assisting someone to die is illegal and punishable by up to fourteen years in prison.

In 2004, noted journalist and social activist, June Callwood, went public about her battle with cancer. Subsequently she also came out in favour of assisted suicide, following the June 2005 introduction of a private member's bill that would legalize it (C-407). June Callwood died on April 14, 2007, at the age of 82.

In 1993, a Canadian farmer, Robert Latimer suffocated his 12 year-old daughter Tracy, who was suffering from severe cerebral palsy and mental retardation. She underwent numerous, major surgical operations to improve her physical condition and was facing another major procedure. In order to save her from more suffering, her father ended her life by hosing the exhaust pipe into his truck with Tracy inside. First Latimer stated that Tracy died in her sleep, but ten days later, when the results from a crime lab changed the focus of the investigation to homicide, he confessed to killing his daughter. A year after Tracy's death, in 1994, Latimer was convicted of second-degree murder. In 1997, after several legal procedures, Latimer was granted constitutional exemption from the minimum sentence of ten years and the judge gave him a two-year sentence. The Crown appealed the sentence and on November 23, 1998, the Saskatchewan Court of Appeal ruled that Robert Latimer must return to prison to serve a life sentence, with no parole for ten years.

The United States

In 1994, Oregon voters approved the "Oregon Death with Dignity Act". The legislative measure made it legal for Oregon doctors to prescribe lethal drug overdoses to terminally-ill patients who ask to die. Oregon became the first and only state in the U.S. to pass such a measure. Because of court challenges, the Oregon Death with Dignity Act (O-DWDA) did not take effect until October 1997.

Since 1998, 171 Oregonians have used the "Death with Dignity" law. The physician is not required by law to be present when the patient ingests the drugs to end his or her life but sometimes the physician opts to be present.

There have been a number of reported legal cases of assisted death in the United States. Ten ended in acquittal, one in a life sentence and the rest in suspended sentences.

The special case of Jack Kevorkian

On June 8, 1990, the *New York Times* reported a doctor who had connected a woman suffering from Alzheimer's disease to a homemade suicide device and watched as she pushed a button and died. It was Dr. Jack Kevorkian who assisted Janet Adkins, who was 54 years old at the time of her death. Her husband, Ronald Adkins said that music was the consuming passion in his wife's life and that when Alzheimer's disease robbed her of the ability to play the piano she no longer wanted to live. Since Mrs Adkins was physically well and her Alzheimer's disease in an early stage, Dr Kevorkian's crusade for doctor-assisted suicide suffered a shaky start. He already had some notoriety by advocating more humane execution of prisoners (Fulton and Metress, 1995).[20] He argued that they should be given the opportunity to choose death by lethal injection coupled with donation of their organs. "The Kevorkian Chronicles" in the cited book, lists dates of assisted suicide and court actions between June 4, 1990 and June 6, 1994 that takes up two full pages.

Dowbiggin states that between 1990 and 1998 Dr Kevorkian

helped 69 people die and only 17 were found to be terminally ill.[21] Support for Kevorkian began to decline towards the end of his career as "Dr Death". He had been charged and tried in three assisted-suicide cases, but juries refused to find him guilty of homicide. Then in the fall of 1998, Thomas Youk aged 52, who was suffering from amyotrophic lateral sclerosis (ALS) asked the doctor to inject him with potassium chloride. Unlike his other cases, Kevorkian himself would inject the lethal dose for the first time. To challenge the laws which forbid mercy killing, Kevorkian videotaped the entire procedure and made the tape available for broadcast on the *60 Minutes* TV program. Charged with first-degree murder, Kevorkian was convicted of second-degree murder and sentenced to 10-25 years in prison. After serving eight years for second-degree murder for his role in one death, he was released from prison on June 12, 2007.

Since 1980 several states have tried to change the law in the USA (Humphry, 2005)[22] including Oregon, Washington, California, Michigan, Maine, Hawaii, and Vermont. Only Oregon has been successful.

The United Kingdom

In September 1992 Dr Nigel Cox, an experienced rheumatologist, was convicted of attempted murder for killing a terminally ill patient who suffered from severe rheumatoid arthritis, was bedridden, had a gastric ulcer and bedsores. All agreed that her life expectancy was very short. Dr Cox openly defied the law and assented to the 70-year-old Mrs Boyes' request for voluntary active euthanasia. Conventional medicine did not relieve the patient's agony. In her last days, when she repeatedly requested to die, the doctor finally gave her an injection of potassium chloride, which ended her life. Dr Cox was found guilty and received a twelve-month suspended sentence. He was also treated with great sympathy by the General Medical Council (the disciplinary body for doctors), and was allowed to continue to practice medicine.

Anthony David Bland (1971-1993) was injured in a soccer stadium disaster in Hillsborough, Yorkshire, UK. He suffered severe injuries that left him in a persistent vegetative state. The hospital, with the support of his parents, applied for a court order allowing him to 'die with dignity'. In March 1993 a Court Order gave permission to let him die. As a result, he became the first patient in English legal history to be allowed to die by the courts through the withdrawal of life-prolonging treatment. The judges said that if he had made a living will expressing his future wishes, he could have been allowed to die in peace earlier.

In the UK, the Assisted Dying for the Terminally Ill Bill was proposed in 2005 to legalise euthanasia and physician-assisted suicide for those with a terminal illness. A House of Lords Select Committee was convened to scrutinize this Bill.[23] The Select Committee did not reach a conclusion on the principle of whether assisted dying or euthanasia should become legal, but identified a number of issues which would need to be addressed in any future legislation.

In May 2006, the House of Lords rejected the Assisted Dying for the Terminally Ill Bill by 148 to 100 votes. The proposer, Lord Joffe, said he would re-introduce the bill.

Scotland

In 1980 the Voluntary Euthanasia Society of Scotland broke away from the English society. From 1992 to 1995 they sponsored research into living wills. In 1996 they also sponsored the University of Glasgow's Research Report on the feasibility of doctor-assisted suicide and an assisted-suicide Bill to be presented to Parliament.

Australia

In Australia it is a criminal offence to assist in euthanasia but prosecutions have been rare. In 2002, police extensively investigated relatives and friends who provided moral support to an elderly woman who committed suicide, but no charges were laid. Nancy Crick was a

69-year-old widow, who had had surgery for bowel cancer and other extensive treatments for the disease. Mrs. Crick claimed to have suffered enough and intolerably and didn't want to live. She killed herself on May 22, 2002 with a powerful barbiturate, surrounded by twenty-one friends and supporters. Her suicide was assisted with drugs by Dr. Philip Nitschke, who in the 1990s championed legislation allowing doctor-assisted suicide in Australia's Northern Territory, and then helped four people to kill themselves before the short-lived law was repealed by the federal government.

Unfortunately, the postmortem examination showed that Mrs Crick was free of cancer but Dr Nitschke—who did not witness the suicide–was not charged by the police.

Germany

Direct killing by euthanasia is a crime in Germany. Interestingly, the country has had no penalty for either suicide or assisted-suicide since 1751.[24] In 2000 a German appeal court cleared a Swiss clergyman of assisted suicide because there was no such offence, but convicted him of bringing into the country the drug that was used.

Italy

In Italy voluntary euthanasia and assisted suicide are forbidden.

Switzerland

In 2001 the Swiss National Council confirmed the assisted-suicide law but retained the prohibition of voluntary euthanasia. A doctor, who out of compassion assists his patient to commit suicide, is not subject to prosecution. Switzerland does not bar foreigners from assisted suicide, but the help must rest on altruistic motives as the law requires. All right-to-die societies are allowed to give help by providing counselling and lethal drugs.

The Netherlands

Both euthanasia and assisted suicide have been widely practised in the Netherlands since 1973 although they were against the law until 2002. The "Termination of Life on Request and Assisted Suicide (Review Procedures) Act" entered into force on April 1, 2002. Dutch law now allows the termination of the life of a patient if the request is voluntary, well-considered, sustained and the suffering is unbearable.

Belgium

The Belgian act legalizing euthanasia was passed in May 2002 and went into effect in September 2002. The Belgian law permits euthanasia and does not define the method.

The only four places that today openly and legally authorize active assistance in dying are: Oregon (since 1997, physician-assisted suicide only); Switzerland (2001, physician and non-physician assisted suicide only); Belgium (2002, permits 'euthanasia' but does not define the method; Netherlands (voluntary euthanasia and physician-assisted suicide lawful since April 2002 but permitted by the courts since 1984).

Euthanasia and public opinion

We have demonstrated through case studies the great diversity of how "mercy killing" is dealt with by many countries. The anguish of the courts and the efforts of the legislators can be seen as they struggle with the complexity of problems that exist under the umbrella of euthanasia.

Yet the disturbing question still lingers and divides opinion on the final judgement of Dr. Kevorkian. Should he be commended for standing up against laws that make dignified death impossible for patients whose remaining life is destroyed by pain and suffering and who want to die? Or is "Dr. Death" promoting something that would inevitably lead society down a path that might end with people being put to death against their will?

In search of an answer, we should consider the views of patients, the public at large and the various ethical and religious concerns about the subject.

There are studies concerning the interest that seriously ill patients have shown in euthanasia and physician-assisted suicide (PAS). An excellent paper in the *Journal of the American Medical Association* (Emanuel et al., 2000)[25] reports on a survey in which only a small proportion of terminally ill patients considered euthanasia or physician-assisted suicide (PAS) for themselves. Over a few months, half of these patients changed their minds. Patients with depressive symptoms were more likely to change their minds about their desire for euthanasia or PAS.

A Gallup Poll in Canada recently showed that 66% of the population gave qualified approval for mercy killing, 24% objected to it and 10% were unsure. The question was formulated this way: "When a person has an incurable disease that causes great suffering, do you or do you not think that competent doctors should be allowed by law to end the patient's life through mercy killing, if the patient made a formal request in writing?" Since 1968 approval of mercy killing has increased from 45% to 66% while disapproval decreased from 43% to 24%.

According to a Gallup Poll[26] the difference of opinion on physician-assisted suicide between religious and non-religious Americans may lie in the fact that this is part of a larger issue concerning the right to die. Defenders of personal liberty maintain that everyone is morally entitled to end their lives when they see fit. For these people, suicide is morally permissible. While suicide in any form is regarded as a sin by many Christians and those of a number of other religions, there is nevertheless a broad range of views among religious Americans.

The Gallup News Service May 17, 2005 reports the latest annual survey on values and beliefs of Americans (Moore, 2005).[27] The survey finds

> that 75% of Americans support euthanasia–allowing a doctor to take the life of a patient who is suffering from an incurable disease and wants to die. But the survey also finds that a much smaller proportion of Americans, 58%, supports doctor-assisted suicide for patients in the same condition.

> The apparent conflict in values appears to be the consequence of mentioning, or not mentioning, the word "suicide".

The latest report from June 2006 confirms the findings of the previous year.[28]

> Gallup's annual survey on Values and Beliefs, conducted May 8-11, 2006, finds that the vast majority of Americans continue to support "right-to-die" laws for terminally ill patients, whether that involves a doctor ending a patient's life by some painless means, or a doctor assisting a terminally ill patient to commit suicide. An analysis of Gallup data collected since 2003 shows that senior citizens, Americans who frequently attend religious services, those with lower levels of education, blacks, conservatives, and Republicans are most likely to object to euthanasia and doctor-assisted suicide.

Most European countries make a distinct category of compassionate murder and permit a substantial reduction in sentences by the courts.

The future of assisted death

It remains problematic whether "freedom from suffering" is a basic human right or not and, if it is a right, what criteria will determine the degree of mild, severe and intolerable suffering. Society, ethics and the law will have to come to a consensus on this

difficult issue, which presently divides not only members of society
at large but also the medical profession, religious thinkers, ethicists
and law makers.

The Canadian Medical Association's policy on Euthanasia and
Assisted Suicide (see Appendix F), is a very thoughtful, unbiased and
forward-looking statement. The policy makes clear the difference
between "euthanasia" and "assistance in suicide". Assisted suicide
means:

> Knowingly and intentionally providing a person with the
> knowledge and the means or both required to commit suicide,
> including counselling about lethal doses of drugs, prescribing
> such lethal doses or supplying the drugs.

As it stands today the clear advice of the CMA is: "Canadian
physicians should not participate in euthanasia and assisted suicide".
Notwithstanding this policy,

> The CMA recognizes that it is the prerogative of society to
> decide whether the laws dealing with euthanasia and assisted
> suicide should be changed. The CMA wishes to contribute the
> perspective of the medical profession to the examination of the
> legal, social and ethical issues.[29]

Concerning religions, there is no fundamental difference between
the Christian and Islamic positions on euthanasia. Neither the
Vatican[30] nor Islamic Law[31] considers euthanasia morally or legally
acceptable.

Nevertheless, there are dissenting views even among Catholic
theologians (Küng and Jens, 1995)[32] and the disagreements remain
unresolved both within the Catholic hierarchy and between the
Catholic Church and other religions.

In 1988, the Unitarian Universalist Association passed a national
resolution affirming the right to die and recently the Knesset in Israel,
which in ethical issues follows rabbinical approval, legislated a
euthanasia bill (Siegel-Itzkovich, 2005).[33]

Maureen McTeer, a Canadian lawyer, in a well researched and
elegantly written volume deals with assisted suicide and euthanasia
(McTeer, 1999).[34] With reference to assisted suicide she states,

I believe that the law—if we decided that assisted suicide and euthanasia are different in practice and legal effect—must consider mental competence as a key factor. As an advocate for greater individual autonomy in health care and related decision-making, I prefer legal recognition for individual choices that ensure that terminally-ill competent Canadians can keep control at the end of their lives.

On the other hand she opposes legalizing euthanasia on the basis that society has an interest in protecting its members from harm including cases when death is inflicted upon them with the purpose of ending suffering. She also emphasizes the interest of children and the physically and mentally vulnerable who need an even stronger protection against killing.

The well-known Canadian ethicist Margaret Somerville opposes any form of euthanasia as she clearly states in the Medical Journal of Australia.[35] She writes:

Physician-assisted suicide and euthanasia are simplistic, wrong and dangerous responses to the complex reality of human death. For physicians to give lethal injections to their patients or to assist them to commit suicide is inherently wrong from the perspective of principle-based or deontological ethics. But even on a utilitarian or situational ethics analysis, it is ethically wrong–the risks and harms outweigh the benefits.

In a forward-looking book written by the director of the Health Law Institute at Dalhousie University in Nova Scotia, we found constructive ideas about what the law should be for assisted suicide and voluntary euthanasia (Downie, 2004).[36] The author argues that the difference between the withholding and withdrawal of potentially life-sustaining treatment is not a sustainable distinction. After expanding on the explanation of the logic of the statement she also considers that most of the concerns commonly held against decriminalizing assisted suicide and voluntary euthanasia, while very serious and legitimate, apply to the withholding and withdrawal of potentially life-sustaining treatment just as much as they do to assisted suicide and voluntary euthanasia.

Among the discussed and important issues Downie analyses the Canadian Charter of Right and Freedoms and concludes (p.144):

> . . . that the section 241(b) of the Criminal Code breaches section 7 and 15 of the Charter and cannot be saved under section 1. The current regime which requires respect for free and informed refusal of potentially life-sustaining treatment made by competent adults and yet prohibits assisted suicide is unconstitutional.

To refute arguments against legalizing assisted suicide, Downie examines the Dutch experience carefully and in detail and summarizes her opinion this way:

> The Dutch experience with euthanasia does not provide convincing evidence to support the claim that if Canada decriminalizes assisted suicide and voluntary euthanasia, Canada will in fact slide to permitting involuntary euthanasia.

We (L.P.I. and M.E.M.) believe that the first step in improving the present difficult situation would be to narrow the focus of euthanasia entirely to "assisted death". This would eliminate ambiguities, and alleviate the sting of certain emotionally charged terms like "mercy killing" and "doctor-assisted suicide" and thus obviate the negative connotations attached to these terms.

At the same time it would be helpful to acknowledge and not ignore that prolonging life burdened with suffering through medical and technological means has created serious problems. To relegate the solution of these to the doctor's conscience or ethical guidelines is simply not possible when the Law allows suicide but criminalizes the prescription of drugs to do it. Common Law is intolerant of certain forms of painless death, while at the same time it allows death by starvation. These excruciating problems demand clear answers from the legal system to help determine the courses of action available to the physician and the family in case of extreme physical or emotional suffering, especially if the patient is incapable of making the choice. Passively doing nothing to prolong life or withdrawing life-support have resulted in criminal charges against physicians; on the other hand, the families of comatose and apparently terminal patients have instituted legal action against doctors and hospitals to make them stop the use of extraordinary life support.

The way out of this ambiguous situation would be the discussion of a legal definition of "End-of-Life Care" which would include Palliative Care and Assisted Death. This approach might define assisted death as an option for the patient for whom palliative care is, or would be, unable to relieve extreme suffering. "Assisted Death" with strict limitations on the demand for assistance and on the doctor's obligation could lead to a better understanding of the problem and would relieve anxiety both for the patients, arising from the fear of imposed decision and the care-givers from the fear of prosecution. A legal definition of the responsibilities of the ethical committees in hospitals and institutions where assisted death can occur would also be a safeguard against abuse.

We are confident that rational discussions, love for our fellow human beings and mature wisdom will help us take the right action and will find a way out of an unclear and disturbing situation.

Notes

1. *The American Heritage Dictionary of the English Language*, 4th edn., (Houghton Mifflin Company, 2004) <http://www.answers.com/topic/euthanasia>, accessed July 20, 2006.

2. Foot, P., Euthanasia in J. Ladd, (ed.), *Ethical Issues Relating to Life and Death* (New York: Oxford University Press, 1979): 14-40.

3. Dowbiggin, I., *A Concise History of Euthanasia: Life, death, God, and medicine* (Oxford: Bowman and Littlefield, 2005): 54-55.

4. euthanasia in *Encyclopædia Britannica* <http://britannica.com/eb/article-9033299>, accessed June 28, 2006.

5. Medina, L., (ed.), *Euthanasia* (Farmington Hills, MI: Greenhaven Press, 2005): 205-215.

6. Humphry, D., Wickett, A., Euthanasia from the Renaissance through the

early twentieth century, in L. Medina, (ed.), *Euthanasia* (Farmington Hills, MI: Greenhaven Press, 2005): 38-46.

7. Dowbiggin, I., *A Concise History of Euthanasia: Life, death, God, and medicine* (Oxford: Bowman and Littlefield, 2005): 31-34.

8. Erdemir A. D., Elcioglu, O., A short history of euthanasia laws, and their place in Turkish law, *EJAIB*, 11, (2001): 47-49 <http://www.eubios.info/EJ112/EJ112F.htm>, accessed August 15, 2006.

9. As in Dowbiggin n. 7: 81-83.

10. Exit International: A peaceful death is everybody's right <http://www.exitinternational.net/>, accessed July 26, 2006.

11. Paris, J., Moreland, P., Assisted suicide is a transgression of divine sovereignty, in L. Medina, (ed.), *Euthanasia* (Farmington Hills, MI: Greenhaven Press, 2005): 130-140.

12. Kamisar, Y., Some non-religious views against proposed "mercy killing" legislation, *Minn Law Rev,* 42(6), (1958): 969-1042.

13. First Do No Harm members support the World Medical Association Declaration of Geneva, 1948 <http://www.donoharm.org.uk/pdf_files/application_form.pdf> accessed July 26, 2006.

14. Editorial. Withdrawing or withholding life prolonging treatment: A new BMA report fills an ethical vacuum, *BMJ,* 318, (1999): 1709-1710.

15. General Medical Council: Withholding and withdrawing life-prolonging treatments: Good practice in decision-making, August 2002 <http://www.gmc-uk.org/guidance/>, accessed June 23, 2006.
The General Medical Council (the GMC) is the regulator of the medical profession in the United Kingdom.

16. Staff Writer, *Chicago Tribune* (June 30, 2006), Doctors' group votes to oppose euthanasia <http://pewforum.org/news/display.php?NewsID=10818>, accessed August 25, 2006.

17. Lovrics P., Euthanasia's never an answer, *CMAJ,* 161(1), (1999): 18.

18. Gorman, D., A morally irrelevant distinction on euthanasia, *CMAJ,* 161(6), (1999): 685.

19. Law Reform Commission of Canada, *Report on Euthanasia, Aiding Suicide and Cessation of Treatment,* Catalogue No. J31-40/1983: 31-35, (Ottawa: Minister of Supply and Services Canada, 1983).

20. Fulton, G. B., Metress, E. K., *Perspectives On Death and Dying* (Boston: Jones and Bartlett, 1995): 187-197

21. As in Dowbiggin n. 7: 136-138.

22. Humphry, D., Assisted suicide laws around the world in *Assisted Suicide* (March 1, 2005) <http://www.assistedsuicide.org/suicide_laws.html>, accessed July 29, 2006.

23. Finlay I. G., Wheatley V .J., Izdebski, C., The House of Lords Select Committee on the Assisted Dying for the Terminally Ill Bill: Implications for specialists, *Palliat Med*, 19(6), (2005): 444-453.

24. Humphry D., Tread carefully when you help to die. Assisted suicide laws around the world (March 1, 2005) <http://www.assistedsuicide.org/suicide_laws.html>, accessed July 29, 2006.

25. Emanuel, E. J., Fairclough, D. L., Emanuel, L. L., Attitudes and desires related to euthanasia and physician-assisted suicide among terminally ill patients and their caregivers, *JAMA*, 284, (2000): 2460-2468.

26. Gallup, Jr., G., H., (Senior Staff Writer) Views on doctor-assisted suicide follow religious lines, (September 10, 2002) <http://poll.gallup.com/content/default.aspx?ci=6754&pg=1>, accessed August 17, 2006.

27. Moore, D. W., The Gallup Poll, from Three in four Americans support euthanasia, (May 17, 2005) <http://poll.gallup.com/default.aspx?ci=16333&pg=1>, accessed August 1, 2006.

28. Carroll, J., The Gallup Poll from Public continues to support Right-to-Die for terminally ill patients, (June 16, 2006) <http://poll.gallup.com/content/default.aspx?ci=23356>, accessed August 1, 2006.

29. Appendix F: The Canadian Medical Association's policy on *Euthanasia and Assisted Suicide* (1998). Issues concerning future perspectives are on pages 2-3.

30. Franjo Cardinal, Seper Prefect, and Hamer, Jerome O. P. Tit. Archbishop of Lorium Secretary, Rome, *The Sacred Congregation for the Doctrine of the Faith*, May 5, 1980.
". . . no one is permitted to ask for this act of killing, either for himself or herself or for another person entrusted to his or her care, nor can he or she consent to it, either explicitly or implicitly, nor can any authority legitimately recommend or permit such an action. For it is a question of the violation of the divine law, an offence against the dignity of the human person, a crime against life, and an attack on humanity."

31. "The Shari'a (Islamic Law) listed and specified the indications for taking life (i.e. the exceptions to the general rule of sanctity of human life), and they do not include mercy killing or make allowance for it. Human life *per se* is a value to be respected unconditionally, irrespective of other circumstances. The concept of a life not worthy of living does not exist in

Islam. Justification of taking life to escape suffering is not acceptable in Islam."
<http://www.islamicity.com/Science/euthanas.shtml#EUTHANASIA%20-
%20MERCY%20KILLING>, accessed August 25, 2006.

32. Küng, H., Jens, W., with contributions by D. Niethammer, and A. Eser, *Dying with Dignity: A plea for personal responsibility*, (J. Bowden, tr.) *Menschenwürdig Sterben. Ein Plädoyer für Selbstverantwortung*, (New York: The Continuum Publishing Company, 1995)

33. Siegel-Itzkovich, J., Knesset passes euthanasia bill from *Jerusalem Post* (December 6, 2005) <http://www.jpost.com/servlet/Satellite?pagename=JPost%2 FJPArticle%2FShowFull&cid=1132475695637>, accessed August 2, 2006.
"The recommendations that formed the basis for the bill were prepared by a 58-member public committee of physicians, scientists, medical ethicists, social workers, philosophers, nurses, lawyers, judges and clergymen representing the main religions in Israel."

34. McTeer, M. A., *Tough Choices: Living and dying in the 21st century* (Toronto: Irwin Law, 1999): 105-130.

35. Somerville, M., "Death talk": Debating euthanasia and physician-assisted suicide in Australia, *MJA*, 178(4), (2003): 171-174 <http://www.mja.com.au/public/issues/178_04_170203/som10499_fm.html>, accessed July 26, 2006.

36. Downie, J. G., *Dying Justice: A case for decriminalizing euthanasia and assisted suicide in Canada* (Toronto: University of Toronto Press, 2004): 87-106 and 144.

CHAPTER 7
LIFE AFTER DEATH

Our concern with life after death

To modern human beings who have witnessed the unprecedented dominance of science over the supernatural, the concept of life after death may appear as an unverifiable assumption. Nevertheless, the human awareness of the inevitability of death generates understandable concern about the sequel to death.

The physical sequel to death is clear from a scientific point of view; the body disintegrates and is reabsorbed into the inanimate component of the biosphere. As Arnold Toynbee summarizes:[1]

> Between the biosphere's inanimate and animate components there is a constant interchange of matter . . . but a live organism does not consist solely of the matter that constitutes the body; it is a specimen of animate matter; and a human being is not only animate; he is also conscious, and his consciousness enables him to make choices, to remember past events, and to foresee some future events, among others, his own inevitable eventual death.

A new, continued or transformed existence after death is a belief which has been found in virtually all cultures. The oldest burials that suggest belief in life after death can be placed in the period between 50,000 and 3,000 BC when corpses accompanied by stone tools, were laid in holes in the ground.

In Hindu mythology, the soul, after death, leaves the body and may go one of two ways: the way of the Gods, which ends in Brahma or the road of the Ancestors, which returns to earth. The belief in transmigration and rebirth is connected to the belief in karma, that is, the function of one's conduct in successive states of existence which determines the fate of one's rebirth.

This ideology of recycling is more prominent in Chinese Buddhism which teaches that the present world, including the universe, goes through a continuous process of creation, duration and destruction. Human beings, depending on their actions, are reborn as gods, humans, animals or tormented spirits. The doctrine of karma is also found in the Buddhist's belief that after death the soul journeys to purgatory where it is judged, punished until the misdeeds of the past life are expiated, and then reborn into circumstances contingent upon the record of the past life.

Ancient Egyptian religion, which covers a time from the Late Neolithic Period to the first few centuries AD, was a blend of folk traditions and the court religions of the Pharaohs, with a strong belief in an afterlife as attested to by the findings in tombs: the dead needed offerings of food and drink. According to these beliefs, a person's spiritual power extends beyond their personal life. There is reference to three kinds of souls: ka, the vital force that outlasts mankind, the bird shaped ba-soul which is set free only after death, and the akh-soul, which can appear as a ghost and ascend to heaven to live among the stars or descend into the underworld. The concept of a judgement was also known and accordingly, Osiris and forty-two judges were to hear the recitation of the uncommitted transgressions by the dead.

In Biblical Judaism, words such as nefesh, neshama and ruah were used, which mean soul or spirit. Human beings were not considered to be dual creatures; they did not possess nefesh, they were nefesh, a unit of vital power and an inseparable entity of body and spirit. During the second century BC, nefesh began to be interpreted as a psychic entity with a separate existence from the body. In Hellenistic Judaism, the influence of Plato, who thought that the soul was imprisoned in the flesh, led to a clear cut dualism. Later, the concept of sheol, the existence of the dead in a shadow of the echo of the living, became the idea of life after death and it was seen as release from the bondage of the body.

The Romans formed a complex and imaginative picture of the afterlife. Their care for the dead was expressed in decorated tombs and lavish sacrifices. Although they believed in the underworld, Hades, they also thought that the individuality of the dead continued and that the dead should take pleasure in their graves so as not to return to haunt the living.

Christian doctrine teaches that there is eternal reward or eternal punishment after the last judgement. The immortality of the soul conquers death. The concept of resurrection, judgement and the immortality of the soul have been elaborated from medieval doctrines with many variations and fragmentations that continue until today. The soul leaves the body and goes to heaven, hell or purgatory, depending on the specific interpretation of a great variety of Christian denominations and sects. Purgatory is a temporary place of punishment where, after suffering and cleansing, salvation is achieved. The mainstream belief of Christianity is that the fate of the soul depends on the faith that Jesus' death has freed mankind from the consequences of sin. This faith, however, according to Christian beliefs, should manifest itself in good deeds as an inevitable sign of its reality. It is possible to make such an act of faith even on a deathbed, in which case the soul may go to heaven without the person having lived in conformity with Christian morality

Islam is best represented by the writings of Avicenna who in the 11th century gave a coherent treatise on body and soul. According to this Iranian physician, the soul is an indivisible, immaterial and incorruptible substance, not imprinted in matter but created with the body which it uses as an instrument. The soul survives and retains all the individual characteristics that it achieved in its earthly existence and, in this sense, it is rewarded or punished for its past deeds.

Concerning the ultimate questions, William James (1842-1910), a pragmatist philosopher and the most influential American psychologist at the beginning of the last century, directly pursued religious experience of the nature of God through psychical research into survival after death. He concluded that survival after death was unproven but, the existence of divinity he held to be established by the record of religious experience.

Julian Huxley (1887-1975) with his scientific humanism eliminated any notion of personal supernatural beings and recognized our phenomenal universe as a system characterized by consistent laws in which human values have no existence outside human society.[2] These values nevertheless are of paramount importance for the life of human beings. Based on human affectivity they are relevant for the regulation of social life. Scientific humanism involves respect for human values such as dignity and individuality, as well as, concern with the aesthetic side of life as reflected in art and literature.

Bertrand Russell (1872-1970), an agnostic, stated that the five ultimate questions which science is unable to answer are: Is there survival after death? Does mind dominate matter or vice versa? Has the universe a purpose? Is there any validity in the assumption of natural law? and What is the importance of life in a cosmic scheme?

If all the variant beliefs and scientific convictions are taken as evidence of our continuous and changing concern with death, one can foresee changes in interpretation of the relationship of mind versus body, mind versus soul and the new scientific interpretation of the existence or non-existence of an afterlife.

Some interesting findings came to relieve the insatiable thirst of readers curious to know about the existence of afterlife in a small book, *Life after Life* written by Raymond Moody, a PhD in philosophy and psychology (1975).[3] This generated an enormous interest in the subject and became in a short time a best-seller. The text is an anecdotal account but provides a useful summary of the **near-death experience (NDE)**.

The near-death experience

Since the 1970s there has been a growing interest in this phenomenon with the assumption that the subjective experience of being close to death would increase human insight into the nature and understanding of the existence of an afterlife. An ever-growing number of books and articles, some involving significant research in terms of numbers and interviews, should attest to this statement.[4, 5, 6]

An overview of the near-death material reveals some interesting findings. The frequency of certain subjective experiences, such as, similar visual, auditory and psychological phenomena, cannot be dismissed as ridiculous and deserve closer scrutiny and critical interpretation (Greyson and Flynn, 1984).[7] This is just one of life's events where the understanding of the concept of brain death should help the rational mind to draw valid conclusions.

Life after Life catalogued the recollections of 150 patients who almost died and were able to recall what they had experienced. He listed the following visions and sensations common to most people who had, what he called, "near-death experience":

- Hear themselves pronounced dead
- Experience unusual auditory sensations (buzzing, ringing, musical sounds)
- Feel themselves moving through a dark tunnel or space
- Separate from their body (floating, detachment)
- See spirits of others
- Encounter a being of light
- Sense a border between two dimensions of existence
- Have a feeling of peace and painlessness

Moody noted that although there were widely divergent circumstances and varying types of persons involved in NDE, there was a uniform pattern of certain experiences. It was suggested that this may have been responsible for the similarities in religious beliefs in cultures separated from each other in time and geographical location (Aries, 1981).[8] There is, unfortunately, a scarcity of quality papers with the methodology suitable to allow scientific scrutiny of some of these conclusions (Siegel, 1984),[9] (Carr, 1984).[10]

The phenomenon is considered to be a fairly common occurrence in modern clinical settings (Lukoff et al., 1998).[11] According to a Gallup poll approximately eight million Americans claim to have had a near-death experience (Mauro, 1992).[12] A recent study attempts to achieve scientific proof of the nature of this phenomenon, but doesn't contribute to the understanding of its nature (Sartori, 2006).[13]

Greyson, who has published about two dozen papers on NDE, has found a variety of references for the study of the phenomenon (Greyson, 2003).[14]

The experience of a close encounter with death is found to include such factors as: subjective impressions of being outside the physical body, visions of deceased relatives, visions of religious figures or beings of light, transcendence of ego and spatiotemporal boundaries, the sense of moving up or through a narrow passageway (tunnel experience), life review, and other transcendental experiences.

In order to bring the pathophysiology of brain death into the interpretation of these phenomena, we shall summarize the somatic sequence of death before we list the nature and frequency of the psychological phenomena described in near-death experience.

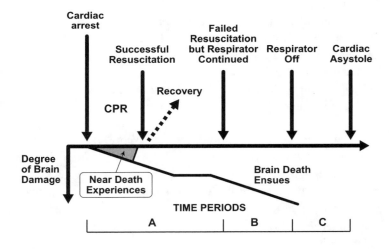

Fig. 5. The near-death experience triangle; A. the time of cardiac arrest and resuscitation; B. time that follows a failed resuscitation with respiratory support and brain death; C. the time between respirator off and asystole. The up-arrow (in time period A) points to the gray triangle where near-death experience must occur. This is a time when the brain and the rest of the body are not dead. If so, how can the brain possibly experience a peek into the realm of the afterlife? This diagram was modified from our original by Dr. John Dosseter.

The somatic sequence of death (Fig. 5) clearly shows that clinical death is "reversible" as long as the brain is not dead, but is capable of functioning, even though consciousness may have been lost, as happens in fainting, cardiac arrest, shock or drowning. These conditions are typical instances when resuscitation can be successful in spite of "clinical death", based on the old cardio-pulmonary criteria (no pulse, no heart beat, and no respiration). Cardio-pulmonary resuscitation and brain-oriented life support, as we have shown earlier, will revive these victims as long as the process of brain death has not gone beyond the limits of brain resuscitation (4-10 minutes, occasionally more in cases of fresh-water drowning).

NDE must occur during the critical four- to ten-minute period, when the brain suffers from a progressive lack of oxygen due either to cardiac or respiratory arrest. Assuming that NDE coincides with this critical time, we might conclude that the near-death experience is the subjective side of cerebral **hypoxia**. That is, the somatic counterpart of the psychological experience is simply the effect of how oxygen deprivation affects brain metabolism and the erratic functions of the neurons.

Let us examine now, in light of the above reasoning, what constitutes the stages of the near-death experience. According to one of the most credible authors (Ring, 1980)[15] the following recollections were recorded by many patients:

Peace and contentment (60%)
Detachment from one's physical body (37%)
Entering the darkness (23%)
Seeing the light (16%)
Entering the light (10%)

There are several possible neurophysiological mechanisms to explain these feelings and visual experiences. Carr in 1984[16] proposed that endogenous hallucinogens (certain behaviorally active **peptides**) play a role in the **agonal state**; this theory was also considered by other authors. These **endorphins**, naturally present, are morphine-like substances capable of producing a feeling of pleasure or well-being, may act through the limbic lobe of the brain, which plays an important part in emotional responses. The hyperactivity of the **limbic system** can produce euphoria and auditory, kinetic and visual **hallucinations**– symptoms very similar to those described with NDE.

We propose the following explanation to understand NDE from a neurophysiological point of view:

1. The triggering mechanism is a progressive ischemic-hypoxic change (decreased blood-oxygen availability) with possible hypercarbia (increased carbon dioxide content in the blood). The feeling of peace and tranquillity is most likely the earliest manifestation of decreased neuronal activity (the way tranquilizers work).

2. As the above chemical changes increase in quantity, the endorphin receptors, which show selective vulnerability to hypoxic changes, react in the limbic system, (euphoria and body separation).

3. With progressive changes, other elements of the brain (cortex, grey matter) become involved and when the visual cortex is affected, "blacking out" will occur (entering the darkness).

4. Further changes cause hyperactivity of the same neurons and visual hallucinations become intensified (seeing the light).

5. In the final stage, just before the midbrain reticular activating system is abolished (ARAS, the system responsible for consciousness), a kinetic hallucination occurs which originates either in the limbic system or in the cerebellum (entering the light).

6. When both the cortex and the limbic system are sufficiently hypoxic, neither consciousness nor recording of events and sensations is possible; the patient will be in deep coma and, in case of recovery, have no recollection of somatic or psychic experience.

We do not think that the phenomena of NDE have anything to do with the afterlife. And a well-known, prolific writer and dissident Catholic theologian is in agreement with this assumption (Küng, 1984).[17] After analyzing the literature about near-death experience Küng concludes:

What then do these experiences of dying imply for life after death? To put it briefly, nothing! For I regard it as the duty of theological truthfulness to answer clearly that experiences of this kind prove nothing about the possible life after death.

All of the somatic and emotional experiences that have been described can certainly originate in the brain, caused by the well-known chemical changes that occur in near-death emergencies. Some of the phenomena clearly fall into the realm of a qualitative disturbance of consciousness called hallucination. As Bonta (2004)[18] states:

> . . . three events might be considered as functional models of each other. **Antagonism** to the recognition **NMDA**-site of the receptor induces dissociative anaesthesia and precipitates Near-Death Experience. **Agonist reinforcement** at the modulatory glycine-site of the receptor counteracts negative symptoms of schizophrenia.

This interesting hypothesis points to the similarities between near death experience, schizophrenic hallucinations and sensory experiences under certain type of anaesthetic agents classified as glutamate antagonists.

The interpretation of these phenomena by the affected brain is the response of a progressively faulty cortex that is still capable of processing these images and feelings according to the culturally conditioned and prevailing systems of beliefs.

The problem of mind, body and soul

Let us take a look at this age-old puzzle and focus our attention once again on what has been learned from this new paradigm which redefines death using brain-oriented criteria. Will this new insight into matters of life and death increase our understanding of what constitutes a person and his or her mind and thus relate to what traditionally is called the soul?

Right at the outset, a variety of concepts confronts the solution for "soul" means different things to different people, as reflected in the ever increasing number of definitions:

1. The immaterial essence of substance, animating principle, or actuating cause of life or of the individual life.
2. The psychical or spiritual principle in general shared by or embodied in individual human beings or all beings having a rational and spiritual nature.
3. The immortal part of man having permanent individual existence contrasted with body.
4. A person's total self in its living unity and wholeness— sometimes distinguished from spirit.

These four definitions come from *Webster's Dictionary* (1976) which lists even more definitions, an indication that compressing the soul into one single sentence remains difficult.[19]

The *Encyclopædia Britannica*[20] defines soul as follows:

in religion and philosophy, the immaterial aspect or essence of a human being, that which confers individuality and humanity, often considered to be synonymous with the mind or the self. In theology, the soul is further defined as that part of the individual which partakes of divinity and often is considered to survive the death of the body.

This means in common usage that the soul is an immaterial principle or aspect that, with the body, constitutes the human person.

In our discussion, we shall consider that the soul is presumably immaterial, that it is immortal, that it is not the same as the mind, and that body and soul together constitute the human person.

The definition of the mind appears somewhat simpler if we accept the premise that the mind is not quite synonymous with the soul. It has a strong identity with the Latin "mens" (as in, *mens sana in corpore sano*: sound mind in sound body) and is synonymous with psyche. The following definition will be adopted for the sake of this discussion:

> in the Western tradition, the complex of faculties involved in perceiving, remembering, considering, evaluating, and deciding. Mind is in some sense reflected in such occurrences as sensations, perceptions, emotions, memory, desires, various types of reasoning, motives, choices, traits of personality, and the unconscious.[21]

Mind therefore is an organized group of activities in the nerve cells in various parts of the brain, in response to the outside world's physical and non-physical events, which the brain has perceived, classified, transformed, and coordinated. The mind initiates actions whose consequences are foreseeable from the already stored and available information.

The definition of body should not present a problem because common understanding and science both agree that body contrasts with mental or spiritual, and that it means the physical substance of a human being or as defined in *Webster's*: "the material part or nature of man".

We shall now examine the evolution of the concept and relationship of the mind/body/soul triad from a historical perspective focussing on what philosophy, religion and science can offer to the understanding of the complexity and interrelatedness of these entities.

The basic meaning of soul in ancient and primitive societies was life. Soul was life and breath, and movement came from the soul. The soul in these archaic views was located variously in the heart, liver or almost any part of the body.

The different concepts of the soul and its relation to the body led to varying developments of thought. Often the soul was regarded as inseparably connected to the body, and was thought to cease at death. Some viewed the soul as a pure and eternal element that attained perfection only after separation from the body at death as in the thought of Plato and Plotinus.

Among Hindus and Buddhists, the soul reincarnates in

successive bodily existences in a recurrent cycle from which release may be obtained through moral, intellectual or spiritual perfection. This dualistic view of body and soul is held by Talmudic Jews and Christians. Jesus made clear the dualistic demarcation between flesh and spirit. St Paul regarded spirit (pneuma) as a divinely inspired life principle, soul (psyche) as man's life in which spirit manifests itself, and body (soma) as the physical mechanism animated by soul. The Stoic philosophers such as Seneca (4 BC-65 AD) held to a dualistic notion, believing that the flesh and soul were in opposition.

Twentieth-century philosophers and scientists have generally followed William James' lead, holding that man is understandable without any recourse to the notion of soul. Sir Russell Brain,[22] an outstanding neurologist, stated in 1961, "we are now, for the first time, beginning to acquire a comprehensive view of mind. We see it inherent in the evolutionary process, growing from elementary beginnings into a subordinate, and finally the dominant factor in evolutionary advance."

The problem, of course, becomes even more complex with the acceptance of evolution as the scientific theory to explain the ascendance of human beings from very modest beginnings to the creature of today. We are now able to manipulate tools and control or destroy the environment by creating more and more complex tools, machines and formidable weapons and to transform the hostile jungle of forests into the hostile jungle of the modern city. If a human body with its brain developed from the body and brain of lower animals, is the same true of the mind? If not, he or she must be qualitatively different from animals and the mind or soul must have been introduced into evolution by some supernatural agency.

Sir Russell Brain, in a chapter on this subject quotes Samuel Butler:

> God makes the grass grow because we do not understand how
> the earth and water near a piece of grass are seized by the grass
> and converted into more grass; but God does not mow the
> grass and make hay of it. As soon as we understand a thing, we
> remove it from the sphere of God's action.

Julian Huxley and Arthur Koestler, two eminent renaissance

men of the twentieth century, adopted scientific humanism as their leading ideology, eliminating any notion of personal supernatural beings and considering the hereafter, and the survival of the body or the soul after death, a case of wishful thinking.[23] Among modern thinkers, philosophers and scientists there is no good agreement about the proper use of the words "mental" and "mind" and, according to Russell Brain, confusion would be reduced by using terms like "subjective experience" and "behavior". Similar confusion exists because of the theological distinction between body and soul. Using "behavior" for a phenomenon which is observed and "mind" for what is subjectively experienced, we can eliminate much of the ambiguity in the meanings. We then can infer the existence of mind in other people from their behavior and be cognizant of our own mind from thinking, knowing, feeling and willing.

Failure of the brain to develop or reconstitute itself after a disastrous insult (massive head injury or stroke) limits the development of the mind or eliminates its achievements. Destruction of the temporal lobe can cause a person to lose his or her memory and destruction of the frontal lobes can cause loss of integration of personality and loss of inhibitions. Memory, feelings and hallucinations, on the other hand, can be elicited by stimulating certain parts of the brain with tiny electrodes (e.g. during surgery under local anaesthesia for the treatment of epilepsy).

There is no doubt that most neuroscientists of today believe that human behavior and subjective experience are clearly and intimately related to the functions of the brain. The mind is the totality of the behaviorally observable functions, whereas the psyche is the totality of subjectively experienced feelings and reflections on the reality of the world, as it appears in the mind of the individual. There is an overlap in what we may call the territorial entities of the mind and the psyche. The deficits of the mind are organically and anatomically more clearly definable than disturbances of the psyche, which are more accessible to biochemical definitions.

There is no evidence to indicate that either the psyche or the mind can exist without functioning material substance. In fact, the evidence is to the contrary and indicates that part of the psyche can be removed by disease or trauma, that the personality and the psyche can be manipulated by drugs and that mental illnesses can be imitated or limited by chemical means.

Therefore, considering the unity of mind, psyche and body, the authors have no hesitation in accepting a monistic attitude and philosophy, whereby mind and psyche are considered the highest functions of the brain. The brain differs from other organs only in the structure and organization of its cellular elements and represents the endpoint of millions of years of evolutionary change with cellular adaptation to environmental stimuli.

The question of how the soul is related to the brain is more difficult to answer because of the various qualities assigned to the concept of soul by most definitions, and because of the greater variety in interpretations of the nature of the soul than in the nature of the mind. The concept of the soul as more encompassing than psyche and mind is more intimately connected with the concept of personhood and consciousness. With its quantitative and qualitative content it is thought to be part of the moral and ethical framework and the whole value system of the individual.

The impossibility of resolving the question of dualism and monism lies in the fact that neither the finite nor the immortal nature of the soul can be proved. However, psyche and mind can be explained entirely by biochemical and biophysical phenomena that occur in and rely on the vastness of the interrelated networks and modular construction of the brain.

From the vantage point of irreversible coma and brain death, we might say with some confidence that, when the brain is destroyed, neither the mind nor the psyche are in existence because these functions are dependent upon the integrity of the organization and functioning of the brain. If the soul is the totality of these functions, it must cease to exist when the brain is destroyed unless we postulate the immaterial existence of the soul.

Since the law is concerned with the person and religion with the soul, the latter can only say that when personhood ceases, the soul leaves the body and we would agree that indeed this is the case. The difference between scientific thinking and religion lies in the interpretation of where the soul migrates after leaving the body. We do not know about heaven, hell and purgatory because they have never been experienced or witnessed by anybody who could tell us what they are like. We know, however, that the soul survives in other individuals in the functions of other brains as memories of behavior, things done, ideas created, harms done, goodness exercised and the brilliance given in certain masterpieces or everyday things. These are well-known human experiences that have been witnessed and this type of survival appears to be the proven example of a person's immortality, which might be referred to as his or her soul.

As long as proof is lacking to verify the immaterial existence of the soul, human beings will search for the meaning of this entity. Although the concept of brain death brings us closer to the understanding of personhood, even maybe to a better definition of mind and body, the soul remains elusive. The best that we can say, which might satisfy both dualists and monists, is that mind and psyche are functions of the brain and that when the brain dies, no evidence of mind and psyche remains. As Pope Pius XII has stated, in irreversible coma the soul already may have left the body. And on this final point both idealist and materialist philosophers should agree.

Notes

1. Toynbee, A., Koestler, A., et al., *Life After Death* (London: Weidenfeld & Nicolson, 1976).
This book is an excellent account of the possibilities and consequences of belief in life after death.

2. Huxley, Sir Julian, (ed.), *The Humanist Frame* (London: George Allen and Unwin, 1961): 13-48.
The introductory chapter also entitled "The Humanist Frame".

3. Moody, R. A., *Life After Life* (Atlanta, GA: Mockingbird Books, 1975).

4. Lommel, P. van, Wees, R. van, Meyers, V., Elfferich, I., Near-death experience in survivors of cardiac arrest: a prospective study in the Netherlands, *Lancet*, 358, 9298, (2001): 2039-2044.

5. Appleby L., Near-death experience: Analogous to other stress-induced physiological phenomena, *BMJ*, 298, (1989): 976-77.

6. Ring K., *Heading Towards Omega: In search of the meaning of the near-death experience* (New York: Quill William Morrow, 1984).

7. Greyson, B., Flynn, C. P., (eds.), *The Near-Death Experience: Problems, prospects, perspectives* (Springfield, IL: Charles C. Thomas, 1984).
This book, the most comprehensive on the subject, contains both scientific and anecdotal material by seventeen authors in twenty-one chapters.

8. Aries, P., *Western Attitudes Toward Death: From the middle ages to the present* (Baltimore: Johns Hopkins University Press, 1974).
An interesting and articulate review of the social history of the subject.

9. Siegel, R. K., The psychology of life after death, in B. Greyson, C. P. Flynn, (eds.), *The Near-Death Experience: Problems, prospects, perspectives* (Springfield, IL: Charles C. Thomas, 1984): 78-120.

10. Carr, D. B., Pathophysiology of stress-induced limbic lobe dysfunction: A hypothesis relevant to near-death experiences, in B. Greyson, C. P. Flynn, (eds.), as in n. 9, (1984): 125-139.
The reference section contains 75 relevant papers from scientific journals.

11. Lukoff, D., Lu, F. G., Turner, R. P., From spiritual emergency to spiritual problem: The transpersonal roots of the new DSM-IV Category, *JHP*, 38(2), (1998): 21-50.

12. Mauro, J., Bright lights, big mystery, *Psychology Today*, July-August, 1992 <http://www.findarticles.com/p/articles/mi_m1175/is_n4_v25/ai_12383217>, accessed July 31, 2006.

13. Sartori, P., A Long-Term Prospective Study to Investigate the Incidence and Phenomenology of Near-Death Experiences in a Welsh Intensive Therapy Unit from International Association for Near-Death Studies, Inc. (May 24, 2006) <http://www.iands.org/research/important_studies/dr_penny_sartori_phd_ prospective_study.html>, accessed July 31, 2006.

14. Greyson, B., Incidence and correlates of near-death experiences on a cardiac care unit, *Gen Hosp Psychiatry*, 25, (2003): 269-276.

15. Ring, K., et al., *Life at Death: A scientific investigation of the near-death experience* (New York: Coward, McCann and Geoghegan, 1980).
An objective, statistical assessment of experiences reported by patients after near-death experience. He concludes "there are many who reported to me,. . . a heightened sense of the spiritual dimension of life. Whatever we may think of the reality of these experiences, they are real in their effect".

16. Carr, D. B., Pathophysiology of stress-induced limbic lobe dysfunction, a hypothesis relevant to near-death experiences in B. Greyson, C. P. Flynn, (eds.), *The Near-death Experience: Problems, prospects, perspectives* (Springfield, IL:

Charles C. Thomas, 1984): 125-139.

17. Küng, H., *Eternal Life? Life after death as a medical, philosophical, and theological problem* (E. Quinn, tr.), (New York: Doubleday, Image Books, 1984): 3-21.

18. Bonta I. L., Schizophrenia, dissociative anaesthesia and near-death experience: Three events meeting at the NMDA receptor, *Med Hypotheses,* 62(1), (2004): 23-28.

19. *Webster's Third New International Dictionary,* Vol. III, (Chicago: G. & C. Merriam Co., 1976): 2176.

20. soul in *Encyclopædia Britannica* (2006) <http://britannica.com/eb/article-9068791>, accessed July 13, 2006.

21. mind in *Encyclopædia Britannica* (2006) <http://www.britannica.com/eb/article-9052811>, accessed July 14, 2006.

22 Brain, Sir Russell, Body, brain, mind and soul, in J. Huxley, (ed.), *The Humanist Frame* (London: George Allen and Unwin, 1961): 51-63

23. Koestler, A., Whereof one cannot speak... ?, in A. Toynbee, A. Koestler, et al., *Life After Death* (London: Weidenfeld & Nicolson, 1961): 238-258.

Journals and abbreviations

Abbreviation	Title of Journals
Am J Dis Child	American Journal of Diseases of Children
Am J Respir Crit Care Med	American Journal of Respiratory and Critical Care Medicine
Ann Intern Med	Annals of Internal Medicine
Ann Neurol	Annals of Neurology
Ann N Y Acad Sci	Annals of the New York Academy of Science
Arch Neurol	Archives of Neurology
Arch Neurol Psychiat	Archives of Neurology and Psychiatry
Arch Surg	Archives of Surgery
BMJ	British Medical Journal
Brain	Brain: A Journal of Neurology
Br Med J Publishing Group	British Medical Journal Publishing group
CJA	Canadian Journal of Anesthesia
Can J Neurol Sci	The Canadian Journal of Neurological Sciences
Chest	Published by the American College of Chest Physicians

Child's Brain	Indexed by PubMed and Medline as Child's Brain
Clin Rehabil	Clinical Rehabilitation
CMAJ (also Can Med Assoc J)	Canadian Medical Association Journal
Conn Med	Connecticut Medicine
Crit Care Med	Critical Care Medicine
Crit Care Nurs Q	Critical Care Nursing Quarterly
Dtsch Arch Klin Med	Deutsches Archive für Klinische Medizine
EJAIB	Eubios Journal of Asian and International Bioethics
Gen Hosp Psychiatry	General Hospital Psychiatry
JAMA	Journal of the American Medical Association
J Am Geriatr Soc	Journal of the American Geriatric Society
JHP	Journal of Humanistic Psychology
J Child Neurol	Journal of Child Neurology
J Neurol	Journal of Neurology
J Neurol Neurosurg and Psychiatry	Journal of Neurology, Neurosurgery and Psychiatry
JR Coll Phys (Lond)	Journal of the Royal College of Physicians (London)
Lancet	The Lancet
Med Teach	Medical Teacher
Med Hypotheses	Medical Hypotheses
MJA	Medical Journal of Australia
Med Klin	Medizinische Klinik (Munich)

Minn Law Rev	Minnesota Law Review
Neurology	Official Journal of the American Academy of Neurology
Neurophysiol Clin	Neurophysiologie clinique/ Clinical Neurophysiology The official journal of the International Federation of Clinical Neurophysiology
Neuroradiology	Official Journal of the European Society of Neuroradiology
N Eng J Med (also NEJM)	New England Journal of Medicine
Palliat Med	Palliative Medicine
Pediatr Neurosurg	Pediatric Neurosurgery
Pediatr Radiol	Pediatric Radiology
Pediatrics	Official Journal of the American Academy of Pediatrics
Reprod Health	Reproductive Health
Rev Neurol	Revue Neurologique
Schmerz	Der Schmerz (Pain)
Science	Science
Transplant Proc	Transplantation Proceedings: An Official Publication of The Transplantation Society
Union Med Can	L'Union Médicale du Canada
Zbl Gesamte Neurol Psychiatr Berlin	Zentralblatt für Gesamte Neurologie und Pschychiatrie Berlin

Glossary of terms

Afferent: pertains to nerve pathways that conduct stimuli toward the brain.

Agonal state: pertains to the condition of agony prior to death characterized by shallow or laboured respiration and biochemical changes in the blood (e.g. acidosis and accumulation of other chemicals including endorphins).

Agonist reinforcement: in biochemistry, describes a chemical substance that reinforces or imitates a physiologic reaction of a naturally occurring substance.

Alpha rhythm: the normal rhythm on the EEG of a person who is awake but relaxed. With closed eyes the frequency is 8-12 cycles per second. Eye opening changes the rhythm to a low voltage 13-30 hertz oscillation, called beta activity.

Alzheimer's disease: is a neurological disorder characterized by slow, progressive memory loss due to a gradual loss of brain cells.

Anencephaly: a lethal birth defect in which a large portion of the newborn's brain as well as the skull and scalp are missing.

Angiography: examination of the blood vessels using x-rays following the injection of a radiopaque substance. Carotid angiography is injection of radiopaque material into the carotid arteries to show blood circulation in the brain.

Anoxia: the absence of oxygen supply to an organ or tissue.

Antagonism: interference in the physiological action of a chemical substance by another having a similar structure.

Apnea: absence or cessation of breathing.

Apoptosis: programmed cell death. The process is governed by chemical signals a given cell receives from its neighbors.

ARAS: Ascending Reticular Activating System, a chain of nerve cells and their connections that are crucial for maintaining the state of consciousness.

Auditory brainstem response (ABR): ABR audiometry is a neurologic test of auditory brainstem function in response to auditory (click) stimuli.

Auscultation: listening to an organ (heart, lung, etc.), as with a stethoscope.

Autolysed brain detritus: liquefied material with debris of brain tissue.

Autolysis: the process of spontaneous disintegration of cells and tissues resulting from the actions of intracellular enzymes.

Axons: a threadlike process of a neuron, especially the prolonged axon that conducts nerve impulses.

Beating heart cadaver: is the descriptive term of a dead body on respiratory support when death was determined using brain-oriented criteria: see also brain death.

Beta rhythm: a waveform on the electroencephalograms having a frequency from 13-30 cycles per second. It is associated with an alert waking state but can also occur as a sign of anxiety or apprehension.

Blood pressure: see systolic pressure, diastolic pressure, mean blood pressure.

Brain death: death established by brain oriented (neurologic) criteria: Irreversible brain damage and loss of brain function, as evidenced by cessation of breathing and other vital reflexes.

Brainstem auditory evoked response or potentials (BAEP) (synonyms: Evoked Auditory Potentials, Evoked Response): the (BAER) test measures responses in brain waves that are stimulated by a clicking sound to evaluate the central auditory pathways of the brainstem.

Brainstem death: synonymous with brain death, with emphasis on the lack of brainstem functions.

Brainstem reflexes: reflex responses that originate in the brainstem (e.g. corneal reflex, pupillary response, respiration, swallowing).

Brain swelling: see cerebral edema.

Cadaver: a corpse.

Caloric stimulation: the absence of eye movement in brain-dead patients is confirmed with cold water stimulation. The ear canal should be irrigated with iced water after the head has been tilted 30 degrees. If brain death has occurred, there should be no deviation of the eyeballs toward the cold stimulation.

Cardiogenic shock: shock due to heart failure.

Cardiocirculatory death: refers to donors who are "non-heart-beating cadavers". In these instances, death is established using the criteria of cessation of heartbeat and spontaneous respiration as opposed to brain death, when death is determined by using neurological criteria and the donors are often described as "heart-beating cadavers".

Cardiopulmonary resuscitation (CPR): to re-establish heartbeat and respiration through external cardiac massage and artificial respiration.

CBF: short for cerebral blood flow.

Cephalic: pertaining to cranial nerves that carry stimuli towards or away from the brainstem through small openings on the skull, (e.g. cranial or cephalic reflexes).

Cerebral blood flow (CBF): is the amount of blood that enters the brain. Blood normally takes up about 10% of the intercranial space.

Cerebral cortex: the extensive outer layer of gray matter of the cerebral hemispheres, largely responsible for higher brain functions, including sensation, voluntary muscle movement, thought, reasoning, and memory.

Cerebral death: a term for brain death used mainly in the 5th and 6th decades of the twentieth century.

Cerebral edema: brain swelling due to increased volume of the extravascular compartment from the uptake of water in the gray and white matter.

Cerebral perfusion pressure: is the net pressure of blood flow to the brain. It must be maintained within narrow limits because too little pressure could cause brain tissue to become ischemic (having inadequate blood flow), and too much could raise intracranial pressure (ICP).

Cerebrospinal fluid (CSF): is a clear fluid that filters from capillaries into the ventricles of the brain and moves slowly into the space under the arachnoid membrane that covers the brain and spinal cord. The CSF is a very pure saline solution which acts as a cushion for the cortex and the spinal cord.

Cervico-medullary junction: the cervico-medullary transition zone is where the brainstem joins the spinal cord.

CMA: Canadian Medical Association.

Cognitive: concerning the faculties of understanding and reasoning.

Coma: a condition of profound unconsciousness caused by disease, poison or head injury.

Coma vigil: the term for a patient who has no meaningful interaction with his or her environment but exhibits sleep and wake cycles (see Persistent vegetative state).

Computerized tomography (CT): an x-ray imaging, computer-assisted method of visualizing structures of the body, as cross-sections.

CPCR: cardio-pulmonary-cerebral resuscitation includes CPR and brain-oriented measures to maintain normal intracranial pressure and adequate cerebral perfusion pressure.

CPR: cardiopulmonary resuscitation.

Cranial nerves: nerves that arise in pairs from the brainstem and reach the periphery through openings in the skull. There are 12 such pairs in human beings.

CT scan (Computer Tomography): a series of X-rays that show the human body in slices.

Cyanotic: affected with cyanosis, a bluish discoloration of the skin resulting from inadequate oxygenation of the blood.

Decerebrate rigidity: in decerebrate, or extensor posturing, the arms are extended by the sides, the head is arched back, and the legs are extended.

Decerebrate: the functioning of the nervous system at a lower brainstem and spinal cord level, manifested as the deepest coma possible without respiratory arrest.

Decorticate: a total absence of functions that originate in the brain cortex. Deep coma in the acute stage; coma vigil in the chronic stage.

Delta activity: refers to brain waves, 3-per-second slow waves seen in deep sleep and in coma.

Dendrites: a branched extension of a nerve cell that conducts impulses from other nerve cells toward the cell body. A single nerve may possess many dendrites.

Diastolic pressure: the blood pressure during the relaxation of the heart muscle. (The lower number of a blood pressure reading).

Diffuse laminar cortical necrosis: generalized destruction of several layers of nerve cells in the gray matter of the cortex.

Diffuse axonal injury: widespread damage of the axons, the processes of the nerve cells that carry nerve impulses in the white matter to other parts of the nervous system.

DNR: do not resuscitate order.

Domino heart transplantation: occurs when one patient undergoes heart-lung transplantation, and his/her original heart is then given to a second heart-transplant recipient. The opportunity for this procedure can occur when the heart-lung recipient's original diagnosis included a primary pulmonary disease, but with a functionally normal-to-near-normal heart. This procedure may be the only opportunity that a critically ill heart transplant candidate may have to receive a donor heart.

EEG (Electroencephalography): electrical signals produced by the brain neurons are picked up by the electrodes and transmitted to a polygraph, to diagnose brain abnormalities (tumor, epilepsy, coma).

Electrocerebral silence: a flat EEG record, that indicates the absence of cerebral activity.

Encephalopathy: organic disorder of the brain.

Endorphins: naturally occurring morphine-like substances in the body that produce a feeling of well-being.

Endotracheal intubation: the placement of a tube into the trachea (windpipe) in order to maintain an open airway in patients who are unconscious or unable to breathe on their own.

Epidural pressure sensor: a sensing device, placed through a burr hole inside the skull, under the bone and above the dura, that senses the pressure intracranially and sends its measurements to a recording device.

Euthanasia: the act of ending the life of an individual suffering from a terminal illness or an incurable condition, by lethal injection or the cessation of extraordinary measures.

Extubation: the process of removing the endotracheal tube from the windpipe following anaesthesia or assisted ventilation.

Fetal position: a position of the body as seen in a vegetative state: the spine is curved, the head is bowed forward, and the arms and legs are drawn in toward the chest.

Flat EEG: electrocerebral silence that indicates the absence of cerebral activity.

Foramen magnum: a large opening in the posterior base of the skull, where the spinal cord connects with the brain.

Foraminal herniation: or foraminal coning: the raised intracranial pressure causes the shift and herniation of the brain into the foramen magnum ('coning') where it damages the lower brainstem and the respiratory centre, often causing respiratory arrest and brain death.

Global hypoxia: oxygen deprivation that affects the entire brain and causes neuronal or axonal damage as in cardio-respiratory arrest, status epilepticus or carbon monoxide poisoning.

Global ischemia: insufficient blood flow to the whole brain often caused by cardiac arrest that may affect selective areas in the cerebrum, particularly the hippocampus (a structure consisting of gray matter under the floor of each lateral ventricle); intimately involved in motivation and emotion as part of the limbic system and has a central role in the formation of memories.

Hallucination: perception of visual, auditory, tactile, olfactory, or gustatory experiences without an external stimulus and with a compelling sense of their reality.

Harvard criteria: the Harvard ad hoc committee, chaired by anesthesiologist Beecher, examined the definition of brain death and published these criteria in 1968.

Hepatic coma: coma caused by the accumulation of waste products due to liver failure.

Holonecrosis: completely necrotic, dead.

Hypoglycemia: low blood sugar.

Hypothermia: an abnormally low body temperature.

Hypovolemic shock: shock due to blood or fluid loss.

Hypoxia: inadequate oxygenation.

Immunosuppressive therapy: the suppression of tissue rejection (i.e. in transplantation) with certain drugs.

Infarction: death to a part of an organ due to the interruption of blood flow to that region.

Infratentorial: a space under the tentorium. Tentorium is a fold of dura mater over the posterior cranial fossa, separating the cerebellum from the basal surface of the occipital and temporal lobes of the cerebral cortex. The tentorium has a medial opening through which the upper brainstem passes and where high intracranial pressure causes the brain to herniate and damage the nerve fibres that carry stimuli towards and away from the brain.

Intracranial hypertension (Intracranial pressure): increase of pressure in the brain.

Intracranial homeostasis: the maintenance of equilibrium inside the skull by adjusting physiological processes; normal blood flow with oxygenated blood, normal intercranial pressure, production and absorption of cerebrospinal fluid.

Intracranial pressure (ICP): the pressure inside the skull. ICP is measured by various methods and instruments in millimeters of mercury (mm Hg). Normally the pressure is less than 15-20 mm Hg.

Intubation: the introduction of a tube into the windpipe to facilitate breathing, as in anaesthesia.

Ischemic: pertaining to absent or inadequate blood flow to an organ.

Isoelectric EEG: a flat EEG record, usually indicates the absence of cortical activity.

Isotope angiography: see Radionuclide imaging.

Isotope test: see Radionuclide imaging and PET scanning.

Limbic system: a group of interconnected deep brain structures, involved in olfaction, motivated behavior, arousal, and various autonomic functions.

Magnetic resonance imaging (MRI): creating images of the brain and other organs by the use of giant magnets and radiofrequency current.

Mean blood pressure: the arithmetic mean of the systolic and diastolic pressure.

Mechanical respirator: ventilating equipment.

Medulla oblongata: the lowermost portion of the brainstem, continuous with the spinal cord, responsible for the control of respiration and circulation.

Metabolic encephalopathy: caused by kidney disease, drug abuse, frequent alcohol use. Symptoms include irritability, lethargy, tremors and depression. Disorientation and coma may develop. Death can occur in severe cases.

Midbrain (synonym: mesencephalon): the middle portion of the brain. .

Mitotic: mitosis is the process by which all cells divide. Mitotic refers to a phase in which the cell's genetic material is split in two.

MRI (magnetic resonance imaging): involves a scanner using strong magnetic fields and radio waves. It collects and correlates deflections caused by atoms into images and offers sharp pictures to show internal bodily structures with great detail.

Myocardial: pertaining to heart muscle.

NDE: near-death experience.

Near drowning: submersion in water with almost fatal outcome, when the victim was saved with cardiopulmonary resuscitation.

Near-death experience: a strange experience reported by some people who have been on the threshold of death.

Necrosis: the death of cells, or part of an organ or severe damage to a tissue (e.g. muscle or bone).

Neuron: A complete nerve cell, consisting of a cell body and its processes (axons and dendrites). The axons form cables that run within the white matter; the cell body and the dendrites are found in the gray matter.

NMDA receptor: a receptor on the cell membrane for the amino acid glutamate (NMDA = *N-methyl d-aspartate*). Activation of NMDA receptors results in the opening of certain ion channels through the membrane of a nerve cell.

NMDA site: the location of NMDA receptors.

Oculocephalic reflex: also doll's eye reflex, is an eye movement to maintain forward gaze in response to neck rotation. It is considered a normal response.

OPTN: Organ Procurement and Transplantation Network.

PaCO$_2$: partial pressure of CO_2 in arterial blood. In the USA the required value to perform the apnea test is PaCO$_2$ 50 mm Hg.

Palliative care: care focused on providing comfort, not cure, in the context of terminal care.

Palpation: a general term used to describe the process of examination of the heartbeat, pulse, abdomen, etc. by means of touch.

Parenchymography: digitised intra-arterial visualization of cerebral circulation by radioisotopes.

Parkinson's disease (PD): is a neurodegenerative disorder that causes slowed movements, tremor, rigidity, and a variety of other symptoms due to the degeneration, or death, of neurons in the brainstem and progressively other areas concerned with movement and other brain functions.

Peptide: a protein-like substance; part of a protein molecule.

Perfusion: the passage of blood into an organ to maintain its viability.

Persistent vegetative state (PVS): is a permanent condition of patients with severe brain damage in whom coma progressed to a state of wakefulness without awareness.

PerVS: persistent or permanent vegetative state.

PET scanning or Positron emission tomography: imaging of the brain by using the positrons of the atom from injected or inhaled radio-active substances.

PVS: persistent vegetative state.

Radionuclide brain scanning: a radionuclide scan is an imaging technique that uses a small dose of a radioactive chemical (isotope) called a tracer that can detect cancer, trauma, infection or other disorders. In a radionuclide scan, the tracer either is injected into a vein or swallowed.

Radionuclide imaging: involves the use of small amounts of radioactive substances to make certain body processes and structures more visible (e.g. circulation of blood in the brain).

Respirator: a programmable machine that maintains artificial ventilation through an endotracheal tube.

Respiratory centre: a group of neurons in the medulla oblongata that integrates sensory information about the level of oxygen and carbon dioxide in the blood and determines the signals to be sent to the respiratory muscles.

Resuscitation: a general term meaning revival.

Scintigraphy: the procedure for obtaining a scintigram, a record of the distribution of a radioactive tracer in a tissue or organ, by means of a scanning scintillation counter.

Senescence: aged, aging process.

Somatosensory evoked potentials (SSEP): are electrical signals generated by the brain to visual, auditory or sensory stimuli (touch, electrical current) and recorded by scalp electrodes. Evoked potentials will be absent in brain death.

Sonography (Ultrasonography): diagnostic imaging in which ultrasound is used to image an internal body structure or a developing fetus.

SPECT (Single-Photon Emission Computed Tomography): a test to evaluate the flow and volume of blood in the brain.

Spinal reflexes: reflexes (e.g. knee jerk) originating entirely in the spinal cord., they may be present in brain death.

Status epilepticus: refers to a life-threatening condition, a state of persistent seizures. It is defined as continuous or recurrent seizures without regaining consciousness between seizures.

Systolic pressure: the blood pressure during the contraction cycle of the heart muscle. (The higher number of a blood pressure reading.)

Tentorial herniation: brain herniation, occurs when a part of the brain pushes downward inside the skull through the tentorial opening, compressing the midbrain and causing neurological signs.

Thalamus: a large ovoid (egg-shaped) mass of gray matter situated in the posterior part of the forebrain that relays sensory impulses to the cerebral cortex.

Ultrasonography: see Sonography.

Uremic coma: coma due to the accumulation of certain waste products caused by kidney failure.

Vegetative state (VS): (also called coma vigil) is the result of traumatic, toxic, or anoxic damage to the brain. It can be transient, of short duration, as well as persistent or permanent. In the vegetative state patients can open their eyelids occasionally and demonstrate sleep-wake cycles. They also completely lack cognitive function.

VS: vegetative state.

Xeno-transplantation: procedure that involves the transplantation of cells, tissues, or organs from an animal source into a human recipient.

Selected Bibliography

BOOKS

Adam, G., *Perception, Consciousness, Memory: Reflections of a biologist* (New York: Plenum Press, 1980).

Adrian, E., Bremer, F., Jasper, H. H., (eds.), *Brain Mechanism and Consciousness* (Oxford: Blackwell, 1964).

Aries, P., *Western Attitudes Toward Death: From the middle ages to the present* (Baltimore: Johns Hopkins University Press, 1974).

Baudouin, J. L., Criteria for determination of death: The approach of the Law Reform Commission of Canada in T. P. Morley, (ed.), *Moral, Ethical, and Legal Issues in the Neurosciences* (Springfield, IL: Charles C. Thomas, 1981): 42-46.

Blank, R. H., Merrick J. C., (eds.), *End-of-Life Decision Making: A cross-national study* (Cambridge, MA: MIT Press, 2005).

Brain, Sir Russell, Body, brain, mind and soul in J. Huxley, (ed.), *The Humanist Frame* (London: George Allen & Unwin, 1961): 51-63.

Bruce, D. A., Coma grading systems and the outcome of coma in L. P. Ivan, D. A. Bruce, (eds.), *Coma: Physiopathology, diagnosis and management* (Springfield, IL: Charles C. Thomas, 1982): 140-146.

Carr, D. B., Pathophysiology of stress-induced limbic lobe dysfunction, a hypothesis relevant to near-death experiences in B. Greyson, C. P. Flynn, (eds.), *The Near-death Experience: Problems, prospects, perspectives* (Springfield, IL: Charles C. Thomas, 1984): 125-139.

Chagas, C., (ed.), *The Artificial Prolongation of Life and the Determination of the Exact Moment of Death* (Citta del Vaticano: Pontifica Academia Scientiarum, 1986).

Davidson, J. M., Davidson, R. J., (eds.), *The Psychobiology of Consciousness* (New York: Plenum Press, 1980).

Dossetor, J. B., *Beyond the Hippocratic Oath: A memoir on the rise of modern medical ethics* (Alberta, Canada: University of Alberta Press, 2005).

Dowbiggin, I., *A Concise History of Euthanasia: Life, death, God, and medicine* (Oxford: Bowman and Littlefield, 2005).

Downie, J. G., *Dying Justice: A case for decriminalizing euthanasia and assisted suicide in Canada* (Toronto: University of Toronto Press, 2004).

Flanagan, O., *The Science of the Mind* (Cambridge, MA: MIT Press, 1993).

Foot, P., Euthanasia in J. Ladd, (ed.), *Ethical Issues Relating to Life and Death* (New York: Oxford University Press, 1979): 14-40.

Fulton, G. B., Metress, E. K., *Perspectives on Death and Dying* (Boston: Jones and Bartlett, 1995).

Furst, C., Consciousness and brain processes in id., *Origins of the Mind* (Englewood Cliffs, NJ: Prentice Hall, 1979): 197-216.

General Medical Council: *Withholding and Withdrawing Life-Prolonging Treatments: Good practice in decision-making* (United Kingdom: The General Medical Council, August 2002).

Greyson, B., Flynn, C. P., (eds.), *The Near-Death Experience: Problems, prospects, perspectives* (Springfield, IL: Charles C. Thomas, 1984).

Guberman, A., Coma as a neurological emergency in L. P. Ivan, D. A. Bruce, (eds.), *Coma: Physiopathology, diagnosis and management* (Springfield, IL: Charles C. Thomas, 1982): 283-317.

Harvey, W., *Exercitatio anatomica de motu cordis et sanguinis in animalibus* (An Anatomical Exercise on the Motion of the Heart and Blood in Animals), (1628).

Hoffman, J., *The Life and Death of Cells* (New York: Doubleday and Company, 1957).

Humphreys, P., Coma in infancy and childhood in L. P. Ivan, D. A. Bruce, (eds.), *Coma: Physiopathology, diagnosis and management* (Springfield, IL: Charles C. Thomas, 1982): 102-125.

Humphry, D., Wickett, A., Euthanasia from the Renaissance through the early twentieth century in L. Medina, (ed.), *Euthanasia* (Farmington Hills, MI: Greenhaven Press, 2005): 38-46.

Huxley, Sir Julian, (ed.), *The Humanist Frame* (London: George Allen and Unwin, 1961): 13-48.

Ivan, L. P., Time sequence in brain death in T. P. Morley, (ed.), *Moral, Ethical and Legal Issues in the Neurosciences* (Springfield, IL: Charles C. Thomas, 1981): 21-24.

Ivan, L. P., Ventureyra, E. C. G., Coma and the evolution of brain resuscitation in L. P. Ivan, D. A. Bruce, (eds.), *Coma: Physiopathology, diagnosis and management* (Springfield, IL: Charles C. Thomas, 1982): 3-16.

Jennett, B., *The Vegetative State: Medical facts, ethical and legal dilemmas* (Cambridge: Cambridge University Press, 2002).

Koestler, A., Whereof one cannot speak...? in A. Toynbee, A. Koestler, et al., *Life After Death* (London: Weidenfeld and Nicolson, 1961): 238-258.

Küng, H., Jens, W., with contributions by D. Niethammer, A. Eser, *Dying with Dignity: A plea for personal responsibility* (J. Bowden, trans.) *Menschenwürdig Sterben. Ein Plädoyer für Selbstverantwortung* (New York: The Continuum Publishing Company, 1995).

Küng, H., *Eternal Life? Life after death as a medical, philosophical, and theological problem* (E. Quinn, trans.) (New York: Doubleday, Image Books, 1984): 3-21.

Ladd, J., (ed.), *Ethical Issues Relating to Life and Death* (New York: Oxford University Press, 1979): 118-145.

Laureys, S., Berré, J., Goldman, S., Cerebral function in coma, vegetative state, minimally conscious state, locked-in symdrome, and brain death, in J. L. Vincent, (ed.) *Yearbook of Intensive Care and Emergency Medicine* (Berlin: Springer, 2001): 386-396.

Law Reform Commission of Canada: *Report on Euthanasia, Aiding Suicide and Cessation of Treatment,* Catalogue No. J31-40/1983 (Ottawa: Minister of Supply and Services Canada, 1983): 31-35.

Lock, M., *Twice Dead: Organ transplants and the reinvention of death* (Berkeley: University of California Press, 2002).

Machado G., Shewmon, A. D., (eds.), *Brain Death and Disorders of Consciousness* (New York: Kluwer Academic/Plenum Publishers, 2004).

Manning, M., *The Hospice Alternative* (London: Souvenir Press, 1984).

McKinney, L. O., *Neurotheology: Virtual religion in the 21st century* (Cambridge, MA: American Institute for Mindfulness, 1994).

McTeer, M. A., *Tough Choices; Living and dying in the 21st century* (Toronto: Irwin Law, 1999): 105-130.

Medina, L., (ed.), *Euthanasia* (Farmington Hills, MI: Greenhaven Press, 2005): 205-215.

Meyers, D., *The Human Body and the Law: A medico-legal study* (Chicago: Aldine Publishing Company, 1970): 139-154.

Moody, R. A., *Life After Life* (Atlanta, GA: Mockingbird Books, 1975).

Nelson, R., Coma in cerebrovascular disease in L. P. Ivan, D. A. Bruce, (eds.), *Coma: Physiopathology, diagnosis and management* (Springfield, IL: Charles C. Thomas, 1982): 126-139.

Ore, G. D., Gerstenbrand, F., Lucking, C. H., *The Apallic Syndrome* (Berlin: Springer-Verlag, 1977).

Paris, J., Moreland, P., Assisted suicide is a transgression of divine sovereignty in L. Medina, (ed.), *Euthanasia* (Farmington Hills, MI: Greenhaven Press, 2005): 130-140.

Plum, F., Posner, J. B., *Diagnosis of Stupor and Coma,* 3rd edn. (Philadelphia: Davis Co, 1981).

Ring, K., *Heading Towards Omega: In search of the meaning of the near-death experience* (New York: Quill William Morrow, 1984).

Ring, K., et al., *Life at Death: A scientific investigation of the near-death experience* (New York: Coward, McCann and Geoghegan, 1980).

Rozovsky, L., *The Canadian Patient's Book of Rights,* rev. edn.,

(Toronto: Doubleday, 1994): 201-209.

Safar, P., Bircher, N. G., *Cardiopulmonary-Cerebral Resuscitation: An introduction to resuscitation medicine*. World Federation of Societies of Anesthesiologists, 3rd edn. (Stavanger: Laerdal, 1988).

Searle, J., *The Mystery of Consciousness* (New York: New York Review of Books, Inc., 1997).

Siegel, R. K., The psychology of life after death in B. Greyson, C. P. Flynn, (eds.), *The Near-Death Experience: Problems, prospects, perspectives* (Springfield, IL: Charles C. Thomas, 1984): 78-120.

Skegg, P. D. G., *Law, Ethics and Medicine* (Oxford: Clarendon Press, 1984).

Supreme Court of the United States, *Cruzan, by her parents and coguardians v. Director, Missouri Department of Health*, 497 U.S. 261, June 25, 1990.

Swanson, J., Cooper, A., *A Physician's Guide to Coping with Death and Dying* (Montreal and Kingston: McGill-Queen's University Press, 2005).

Tooley, M., Decision to terminate life and the concept of person in J. Ladd, (ed.), *Ethical Issues Relating to Life and Death* (New York: Oxford University Press, 1979): 62-93.

Toynbee, A., Koestler, A., et al., *Life After Death* (London: Weidenfeld & Nicolson, 1976).

Veatch, R. M., *Medical Ethics* 2nd edn. (Boston: Jones and Bartlett, 1997).

Veatch, R. M., *Death, Dying and the Biological Revolution: Our last quest for responsibility*, rev. edn., (New Haven: Yale University Press, 1989).

Walker, E., Respirator brain in id., *Cerebral Death* (Dallas: Professional Information Library, 1977): 114-118.

JOURNALS

Addington-Hall, J. M., Karlsen, S., A national survey of health professionals and volunteers working in voluntary hospices in the UK, II, *Palliat Med,* 19(l), (2005): 49-57.

Annas, G. J., "Culture of Life" Politics at the Bedside: The case of Terri Schiavo, N *Eng J Med,* 352, (2005): 1710-1715.

Appleby, L., Near-death experience: Analogous to other stress induced physiological phenomena, *BMJ,* 298, (1989): 976-77.

Arts, W. F. M., Van Dongen, H. R., et al., Unexpected improvement after prolonged post traumatic vegetative state, *J Neurol Neurosurg and Psychiatry,* 48, (1985): 1300-1303.

Asch, D. A., Hansen-Flaschen, J., Lanken, P. N., Decision to limit or continue life-sustaining treatment by critical care physicians in the United States: Conflicts between physician's practices and patient wishes, *Am J Respir Crit Care Med,* 151, (1995): 288-292.

Baumgartner, H., Gerstenbrand, F., Diagnosing brain death without a neurologist, *BMJ,* 324(7352), (2002): 1471-1472.

Berger, E., Vavrick, K., Hochgatterer, P., Vigilance scoring in children with acquired brain injury: Vienna Vigilance Score in comparison with usual coma scales, *J Child Neurol,* 16(4), (2001): 236-40.

Bonta, I. L., Schizophrenia, dissociative anesthesia and near-death experience; three events meeting at the NMDA receptor, *Med Hypotheses,* 62, (2004): 23-28.

Cairns, H., Oldenfield, R. C., Pennybacker, J. B., et al., Akinetic mutism with an epidermoid cyst of the third ventricle, *Brain,* 64, (1941): 273-290.

Canadian Neurocritical Care Group, Guidelines for the diagnosis of brain death, *Can J Neurol Sci,* 26, (1999): 64-66.

Capron, A. M., Brain Death: Well settled yet still unresolved (Editorial), N *Eng J Med,* 344, (2001): 1244-1246.

Chang, M., McBride, L., Ferguson, M., Variability in brain death declaration practices in pediatric head trauma patients, *Pediatr Neurosurg,* 39, (2003): 7-9.

Charatan, F., President Bush and Congress intervene in "right to die" case, *BMJ*, 330, (2005): 687.

Demetriades, D., Kuncir, E., et al., Outcome and prognostic factors in head injuries with an admission Glasgow Coma Scale score of 3, *Arch Surg*, 139(10), (2004): 1066-1068.

Didion, J., The case of Theresa Schiavo, *The New York Review of Books* , Vol. LII, No 10. (June 9, 2005,).

Dillon, W. P., Lee, R. V., Tronolone, M. J., et al., Life support and maternal brain death during pregnancy, *JAMA*, 248, (1982): 1089-1091.

Dragand, A., Grahovac, D. S., Brain death in Croatia, abstract from *The 2nd International Symposium on Brain Death, Havana, Cuba*, (February 2-March 1,1996).

Editorial. Withdrawing or withholding life prolonging treatment: A new BMA report fills an ethical vacuum, *BMJ*, 318, (1999): 1709-1710.

Editorial. The sacred and the secular: the life and death of Terri Schiavo, *CMAJ*, 172(9), (2005): 1149.

Emanuel, E. J., Fairclough, D. L., Emanuel, L. L., Attitudes and desires related to euthanasia and physician-assisted suicide among terminally ill patients and their caregivers, *JAMA*, *284*, (2000): 2460-2468.

Feinberg, W. M., Ferry, P. C., A fate worse than death. The persistent vegetative state in childhood, *Am J Dis Child*, 38(2), (1984): 128-30.

Field, D. R., Gates, E. A., Creasy, R. K., et al., Maternal brain death during pregnancy: Medical and ethical issues, *JAMA*, 260, (1988): 816-822.

Finlay, I. G., Wheatley, V. J., Izdebski, C., The House of Lords Select Committee on the Assisted Dying for the Terminally Ill Bill: Implications for specialists, *Palliat Med*, 19(6), (2005): 444-453.

Fischer, C., The use of EEG in the diagnosis of brain death in France, *Neurophysiol Clin*, 27(5), (1997): 373-382.

Fischer, J., Mathieson, C., The history of the Glasgow Coma Scale:

Implications for practice, *Crit Care Nurs*, 23(4), (2001): 52-58.

Frank, L. M., Furgiuele, T. L., Etheridge, Jr., J. E., Prediction of chronic vegetative state in children using evoked potentials, *Neurology*, 35, (1985): 931-934.

Goodman, M. D., Tarnoff, M., Slotman, G. J., Effect of advance directives on the management of elderly critically ill patients, *Crit Care Med*, 26, (1998): 701-704.

Gorman, D., A morally irrelevant distinction on euthanasia, *CMAJ*, 161(6), (1999): 685.

Greyson, B., Incidence and correlates of near-death experiences on a cardiac care unit, *Gen Hosp Psychiatry*, 25, (2003): 269-276.

Hansotia, P. L., Persistent vegetative state. Review and report of electrodiagnostic studies in eight cases, *Arch Neurol*, 42, (1985): 1048-1052.

Haupt, W. F., Rudolf, J., European Brain Death Codes: A Comparison of National Guidelines, *J Neurol*, 246(6), (1999): 432-437.

Higashi, K., Hatano, M., Abiko, S., et al., Five year follow-up study of the patients with persistent vegetative state, *J Neurol Neurosurg and Psychiatry*, 44, (1981): 552-554.

Hoffmann, J. C., Wenger, N. S., Davis, R. B., et al., Patient preferences for communication with physicians about end-of-life decisions, *Ann Intern Med*, 127, (1997): 1-12.

Huet, H., Leroy, G., Toulas, P., Coskun, O., Theron, J., Radiological confirmation of brain death: digitised cerebral parenchymography. Preliminary report, *Neuroradiology*, 38, Suppl. I, (1996): S42-46.

Hyland, D. K., Dodek, P., Rocker, G., et al., What matters most in end-of-life care: perceptions of seriously ill patients and their family members, *CMAJ*, 174(5), (2006): 627-633.

Ingvar, D. H., Brun, A., Johansson, L., Samuelsson, S. M., Survival after severe cerebral anoxia with destruction of the cerebral cortex: the apallic syndrome, *Ann NY Acad Sci*, 315, (1978): 184-214.

Ivan, L. P., Irreversible brain damage and related problems: Pronouncement of death, *J Am Geriatr Soc*, 18, (1970): 816-822.

Ivan, L. P., Ventureyra, E. C. G., Choo, S., Intracranial pressure monitoring with the fiber optic transducer in children, *Child's Brain*, 7, (1980): 303-313.

Ivan, L. P., Spinal reflexes in cerebral death, *Neurology*, 23, (1973): 650-652.

Ivan, L. P., The persistent vegetative state, *Transplant Proc*, 22, (1990): 993-994.

Jennett, B., Plum, F., Persistent vegetative state after brain damage: A syndrome in search of a name, *Lancet*, 1, (1972): 734-737.

Jennett, B., Brainstem death defines death in law, *BMJ*, 318, (1999): 1755.

Kamisar, Y., Some non-religious views against proposed "mercy killing" legislation, *Minn Law Rev*, 42(6), (1958): 969-1042.

Kinney, H. C., Korein, J., Panigrahy, et al., Neuropathological findings in the brain of Karen Ann Quinlan: The role of the thalamus in persistent vegetative state, *N Eng J Med*, 330, (1994): 1470-1475.

Korein, J., Brain death: Interrelated medical and social issues. Terminology, definitions, and usage. *Ann N Y Acad Sci*, 315, (1978, Nov 17): 6-18.

Kretschmer, E., Das apallische Sydrom, *Zbl Gesamte Neurol Psychiatr Berlin*, 169, (1940): 576-579.

Lazar, N. M., Shemie, S., Webster, G. C., Dickens, B. M., Bioethics for clinicians: 24. Brain death, *CMAJ*, 20, (2001): 164.

Levy, D. E., Knill-Jones, R. P., Plum, F., The vegetative state and its prognosis following nontraumatic coma, *Ann NY Acad Sci*, 315, (1978): 293-306.

Levy, D. E., Sidtis, J. J., Rottenberg, D. A., et al., Differences in cerebral blood flow and glucose utilization in vegetative versus locked-in patients, *Ann Neurol*, 22, (1987): 673-682.

Lloyd-Williams, M., MacLeod, R. D., A systematic review of teaching and learning in palliative care within the medical undergraduate curriculum, *Med Teach*, 26, (2004): 683-690.

Lombardi, F., Taricco, M., De Tanti, A., et al., Sensory stimulation of brain-injured individuals in coma or vegetative state: Results of a Cochrane systematic review, *Clin Rehabil*, 16(5), (2002): 464-472.

Lommel, P. van, Wees, R. van, Meyers, V., Elfferich, I., Near-death experience in survivors of cardiac arrest: A prospective study in the Netherlands, *Lancet*, 358, 9298, (2001): 2039-2044.

Lovrics, P., Euthanasia's never an answer, *CMAJ,* 16(1), (1999): 18.

Lukoff, D., Lu, F., G., Turner, R. P., From spiritual emergency to spiritual problem: The transpersonal roots of the new DSM-IV category, *JHP*, 38(2), (1998): 21-50.

Magoun, H. W., An ascending reticular activating system in the brainstem, *Arch Neurol Psychiat*, 67, (1952): 145-154.

Mollaret, P., Goulon, M., Le coma dépassé, *Rev Neurol* 101, (1959): 5-15.

Multi-Society Task Force on PVS. Medical aspects of the persistent vegetative state, *New Engl J Med*, 330, (1994): 1499-1508.

Nelson, K. R., Lee, S. A., Schmidt, F. A., Does the arousal system contribute to near death experience?, *Neurology*, 66, (2006): 1003-1009.

Owen, A., Coleman, M., Boly, M. et al., Detecting awareness in the vegetative state, *Science*, 313(5792), (September 8, 2006): 1402.

Paris, J. J., The six million dollar woman, *Conn Med*, 45, (1981): 720-721.

Pope Pius XII. The Prolongation of Life: Allocution to the International Congress of Anesthesiologists, November 24, 1957, in *The Pope Speaks,* Vol. 4, (1958): 393-398.

Position of the American Academy of Neurology on certain aspects of the care and management of the persistent vegetative state patient. Adopted by the Executive Board, American Academy of Neurology, April 21, 1988, Cincinnati, OH, *Neurology,* 39(1), (1989): 125-126.

Powner, D. J., Bernstein, I. M., Extended somatic support for pregnant women after brain death, *Crit Care Med*, 31, (2003): 1241-1249.

Powner, D. J., Hernandez, M., Rives, T., Variability among hospital policies for determining brain death in adults, *Crit Care Med*, 32, (2004): 1284-1288.

Quill, T. E., Terri Schiavo: A tragedy compounded, *N Engl J Med*, 352, (2005): 1630-1633.

Report of the Ad Hoc Committee of the Harvard Medical School to examine the definition of brain death. A definition of irreversible coma, *JAMA*, 205, (6), (1968): 337-340.

Rosenberg, G. A., Johnson, S. F., Brenner R. P., Recovery of cognition after prolonged vegetative state, *Ann Neurol*, 2, (1977): 167-168.

Rosenblath, W., Über einen bemerkenswerten Fall von Hirnerschütterung, *Dtsch Arch Klin Med*, 64, (1899): 406-429.

Sabatowski, R., Radbruch, L., Nauck, F., et al., Development and state of the in-patient palliative care institutions in Germany, *Schmerz*, 15, (2001): 312-319.

Safar, P., On the history of modern resuscitation, *Crit Care Med*, 24, (2 suppl.) (1996): S3-S11.

Safar, P., (ed.), Brain resuscitation, *Crit Care Med, Special Issue*, 6, (1978): 199-291.

Seely, J. F., Mount, B. M., Palliative medicine and modern technology, *CMAJ*, 161(9), (1999): 1120-1121.

Sheehy, E., Conrad, S. L., Brigham, L E., et al., Estimating the number of potential organ donors in the United States, *N Engl J Med*, 349, (2003): 667-674.

Shemie, S. D., Variability of brain death practices. Letters to the Editor., *Crit Care Med*, 12, (2004): 2564-2565.

Shemie, S. D., Baker, A. J., Knoll, G., et al., Donation after cardiocirculatory death in Canada: National recommendations for donation after cardiocirculatory death, *CMAJ*, 175(8), (2006): S1-S34.

Shemie, S. D., Doig, C., Belitsky, P., Advancing toward a modern death: The path from severe brain injury to neurological determination of death, *CMAJ*, 168(8), (2003): 993-995.

Shemie, S. D., Doig, C., Dickens, B., et al., Severe brain injury to neurological determination of death: Canadian forum recommendations, *CMAJ*, 174(6), Suppl. (2006): S1-S12. The full text of the document is accessible on the internet : <http://www.cmaj.ca/cgi/content/full/174/6/S1>.

Shemie, S. D., Ross, H., Pagliarello, J., et al., Organ donor management in Canada: Recommendations of the forum on medical management to optimize donor organ potential, *CMAJ*, 174(6), Suppl., (2006): S13-S23.

Souza, J. P., Oliveira-Neto, A., Surita, F. G., et al., The prolongation of somatic support in a pregnant women with brain death: A case report, *Reprod Health*, 3, (2006): 3.

Shuttleworth, E., Recovery to social and economic independence from prolonged postanoxic vegetative state, *Neurology*, 33, (1983): 372-374.

Steinhauser, K. E., Christakis, N., Clipp, E., et al., Factors considered important at the end of life by patients, family, physicians, and other care providers, *JAMA*, 284, (2000): 2476-2482.

Swash, M., Brain death: Still-unresolved issues worldwide, *Neurology*, 58, (2002): 9-10.

Teasdale, G., Jennett, B., Assessment of coma and impaired consciousness: A practical scale, *Lancet*, 2, (1974): 81-84.

Thomke, F., Weilemam, L. S., Current concepts in diagnosing brain death in Germany [article in German], *Med Klin (Munich)*, 95(2), (2000): 95-99.

Ventureyra, E. C. G., Ivan, L. P., Brain resuscitation (special communication), *Can J Neurol Sci*, 6, (1979): 71-72.

Wijdicks, E., The diagnosis of brain death, *N Engl J Med*, 344, (2001): 1215-1221.

Wijdicks, E., Brain death worldwide: Accepted fact but no global consensus in diagnostic criteria, *Neurology*, 56, (2002): 20-25.

Wood, K. E., Becker, B. N., McCartney, J. G., et al., Care of the potential organ donor, *N Engl J Med*, 351, (2004): 2730-2739.

Young, B., Shemie, S., Doig, C., Teitelbaum, J., Brief review: The role of ancillary tests in the neurological determination of death, *CJA*, 53, (2006): 620-627.

Young, K. W., Phelan, R. A., Lehman, J. W., et al., Computed tomographic findings in akinetic mutism, *Am J Dis Child*, 138, (1984): 166-167.

Zegers de Beyl, D., Brunko, E., Prediction of chronic vegetative state with somatosensory evoked potentials, *Neurology*, 36, (1986): 134.

INTERNET RESOURCES

Anon., Abstracts of the 2nd International Symposium On Brain Death, Havana, Cuba (February 27-March 1, 1996) <http://www.changesurfer.com/BD/1996/1996Abstracts.html>, accessed July 20, 2006.

Blizzard, R., The Gallup Poll "Right to Die or Dead to Rights?" (June 5, 2002) <http://poll.gallup.com/content/default.aspx?ci=6265&pg=1>, accessed August 15, 2006.

Byrne, P., Coimbra, C. G., Spaeman, R., Wilson, M. A., "Brain death" is not death! Essay at a meeting of the Pontifical Academy of Sciences in early February. Dr. Paul Byrne to Compassionate Healthcare Network, March 29, 2005 via e-mail <http://www.chninternational.com/brain_death_is_not_death_byme_paul_md.html>, accessed June 8, 2006.

Canadian Council for Donation and Transplantation <http://www.ccdt.ca/english/about/council.html>, accessed April 4, 2007.

cardiopulmonary resuscitation from *Encyclopædia Britannica* <http://www.britannica.com/eb/article-9020301>, accessed May 16, 2006.

Carroll, J., The Gallup Poll from Public continues to support Right-to-Die for terminally ill patients (June 16, 2006) <http://poll.gallup.com/content/default.aspx?ci=23356&pg=1>, accessed August 1, 2006.

China's first brain death standard approved <http://www/china.org.

cn/english/2004/May/94597.htm>, accessed May 28, 2006.

coma from *Encyclopædia Britannica* <http://www.britannica.com/ eb/article-9024905>, accessed April 15, 2006.

Conigliaro, M., Abstract Appeal, Schiavo <http://abstractappeal. com/schiavo/infopage.html>, accessed June 21, 2006.

consciousness from *Encyclopædia Britannica* <http://www. britannica.com/eb/article-9025930>, accessed May 16, 2006.

death in *Encyclopædia Britannica* <http://www.britannica.com/eb/ article-22180>, accessed June 13, 2006.

diving reflex in The American Heritage Dictionaries <http://www.answers. com/topic/mammalian-diving-reflex>, accessed April 26, 2006.

euthanasia in *Encyclopædia Britannica* <http://britannica.com/eb/ article-9033299>, accessed June 28, 2006.

Erdemir, A. D., Elcioglu, O., A short history of euthanasia laws and their place in Turkish law, *EJAIB,* 11, (2001): 47-49 <http:// www2.unescobkk.org/eubios/EJ112/ej112f.htm>, accessed August 15, 2006.

Exit International: A peaceful death is everybody's right <http://www. exitinternational.net/>, accessed July 26, 2006.

Fins, J. J., Schiff, N. D., In Brief: The afterlife of Terri Schiavo. *The Hastings Center Report* (2005) <http://www.medscape.com/ viewarficles/511647>, accessed June 24, 2006.

First Do No Harm members support the World Medical Association Declaration of Geneva, 1948 <http://www.donoharm.org.uk/ pdffiles/applicationform.pdf>, accessed July 26, 2006.

Freer, J., Ethics Committee Core Curriculum, Online Edition, Brain Death UB Center for Clinical Ethics and Humanities in Health Care <http://wings.buffalo.edu/faculty/research/bioethics/man-deth. html>, accessed August 24, 2006.

Gallup, Jr., G. H., (Senior Staff Writer) Views on doctor-assisted suicide follow religious lines (September 10, 2002) <http://poll. gallup.com/content/default.aspx?ci=6754&pg=1>, accessed August 17, 2006.

General Medical Council: Withholding and withdrawing life-prolonging treatments: Good practice in decision-making (August 2002) <http://www.gmc-uk.org/guidance/>, accessed June 23, 2006.

Humphry D., Tread carefully when you help to die. Assisted suicide laws around the world (March 1, 2005) <http://www.assistedsuicide.org/suicide_laws.html>, accessed July 29, 2006.

Jorgensen, E. O., Two standards of death in Denmark. Death in Denmark is either cardiac death or brain death. The 2nd International Symposium on Brain Death, Havana, Cuba, (February 27-March 1, 1996) [abstract] <http://www.changesurfer.com/BD/1996/1996Abstracts.html>, accessed August 3, 2006.

Kuchta, J., 55. Jahrestagung der Deutschen Gesellschaft für Neurochirurgie e.V. (DGNC), from Brain death versus brainstem death: An international analysis of historic and actual criteria to diagnose death <http://www.egms.de/en/meetings/dgnc2004/04dgnc0147.shtml>, accessed August 8, 2006.

Mauro, J., Bright lights, big mystery, *Psychology Today*, July-August, 1992 <http://www.findarticles.com/p/articles/mi_m1175/is_n4_v25/ai_12383217>, accessed July 31, 2006.

May, W. E., Caring for persons in the "persistent vegetative state" and Pope John Paul II's March 20, 2004 address "On life sustaining treatments and the vegetative state", (October 23, 2005) <http://www.christendom-awake.org/pages/may/caringforpersons.html>, accessed June 24, 2006.

mind in *Encyclopædia Britannica* <http://www.britannica.com/eb/article-9052811>, accessed July 14, 2006.

Moore, D. W., The Gallup Poll from Three in four Americans support euthanasia (May 17, 2005) <http://poll.gallup.com/default.aspx?ci=16333&pg=1>, accessed August 1, 2006.

Moore, D. W., Public supports removal of feeding tube for Terri Schiavo, *Gallup News Service*, (March 22, 2005) <http://poll.gallup.com/content/default.aspx?ci=15310&pg=1&VERSION=p>, accessed June 23, 2006.

Morioka, M., Reconsidering brain death: A lesson from Japan's fifteen years of experience, *Hastings Center Report*, 31, no. 4, (2001) <http://www.lifestufies.org/reconsidering.html>, accessed June 23, 2006.

Pataki, Governor George, New York State Task Force on Life and the Law <http://www.health.state.ny.us/nysdoh/consumer/patient/chap5.htm>, accessed April 30, 2006.

Pope Paul II declares feeding tube removal immoral. Right to Life Committee Spring/Summer 2004. IRLC News <http://www.illinoisrighttolife.org/2004_2FeedingTubeRemovalImmoral.html>, accessed June 24, 2006.

Resuscitation from Royal Humane Society <http://www.scholarly-societies.org/history/1774rhs.html>, accessed August 20, 2006.

Sachedina, Abdulaziz, Brain Death in Islamic Jurisprudence <http://www.people.virginia.edu/~aas/article/article6.htm>, accessed June 28, 2006.

Sartori, P., A Long-Term Prospective Study to Investigate the Incidence and Phenomenology of Near-Death Experiences in a Welsh Intensive Therapy Unit from International Association for Near-Death Studies, Inc. (May 24, 2006) <http://www.iands.org/research/important_studies/dr_penny_sartori_phd_prospective_study.html>, accessed July 31, 2006.

Shemie, S. D., Doig, C., Dickens, B., et al., Severe brain injury to neurological determination of death: Canadian forum recommendations, *CMAJ*, 174(6), Suppl. (2006): S1-S12 <http://www.cmaj.ca/cgi/content/full/174/6/S1>, accessed June 2007.

Siegel-Itzkovich, J., Knesset passes euthanasia bill from *Jerusalem Post* (December 6, 2005) <http://www.jpost.com/servlet/Satellite?pagename=JPost%2FJPArticle%2FShowFull&cid=11324756956 37>, accessed August 2, 2006.

Somerville, M., "Death talk": Debating euthanasia and physician-assisted suicide in Australia, *MJA*, 178(4), (2003): 171-174 <http://www.mja.com.au/public/issues/178_04_170203/som10499_fm.html>, accessed July 26, 2006.

soul in *Encyclopædia Britannica* <http://britannica.com/eb/article-9068791>, accessed July 13, 2006.

Staff Writer, *Chicago Tribune* June 30, 2006: Doctors group votes to oppose euthanasia <http://pewforum.org/news/display.php?NewsID=10818>, accessed August 25, 2006.

Appendix A

World Medical Association Declaration on Death

Adopted by the 22nd World Medical Assembly Sydney, Australia, August 1968, as amended by the 35th World Medical Assembly Venice, Italy, October 1983.

The determination of the time of death is in most countries the legal responsibility of the physician and should remain so. Usually the physician will be able without special assistance to decide that a person is dead, employing the classical criteria known to all physicians.

Two modern practices in medicine, however, have made it necessary to study the question of the time of death further:

1. the ability to maintain by artificial means the circulation of oxygenated blood through tissues of the body which may have been irreversibly injured and
2. the use of cadaver organs such as heart or kidneys for transplantation.

A complication is that death is a gradual process at the cellular level with tissues varying in their ability to withstand deprivation of oxygen. But clinical interest lies not in the state of preservation of isolated cells but in the fate of a person. Here the point of death of the different cells and organs is not so important as the certainty that the process has become irreversible by whatever techniques of resuscitation that may be employed.

It is essential to determine the irreversible cessation of all functions of the entire brain, including the brainstem. This determination will be based on clinical judgment supplemented if necessary by a number of diagnostic aids. However, no single technological criterion is entirely satisfactory in the present state of medicine nor can any one technological procedure be substituted for the overall judgment of the physician. If transplantation of an organ is involved, the decision that death exists should be made by two or more physicians and the physicians determining the moment of death should in no way be immediately concerned with performance of transplantation.

Determination of the point of death of the person makes it ethically permissible to cease attempts at resuscitation and in countries where the law permits, to remove organs from the cadaver provided that prevailing legal requirements of consent have been fulfilled.

Appendix B

Diagnosis of Death in U. K.

Memorandum issued by the honorary secretary of the Conference of Medical Royal Colleges and their Faculties in the United Kingdom on 15 January 1979

Printed with permission of the BMJ Publishing Group.

British Medical Journal, 1979, Feb 3: 1(6159): 332

(1) In October 1976 the Conference of Royal Colleges and their Faculties (UK) published a report[1,2] unanimously expressing the opinion that "brain death", when it had occurred, could be diagnosed with certainty. The report has been widely accepted. The conference was not at that time asked whether or not it believed that death itself should be presumed to occur when brain death takes place or whether it would come to some other conclusion. The present report examines this point and should be considered as an addendum to the original report.

(2) Exceptionally, as a result of massive trauma, death occurs instantaneously or near-instantaneously. Far more commonly, death is not an event: it is a process, the various organs and systems supporting the continuation of life failing and eventually ceasing altogether to function, successively and at different times.

(3) Cessation of respiration and cessation of the heartbeat are examples of organic failure occurring during the process of dying, and since the moment that the heartbeat ceases is usually detectable

with simplicity by no more than clinical means, it has for many centuries been accepted as the moment of death itself, without any serious attempt being made to assess the validity of this assumption.

(4) It is now universally accepted, by the public as well as by the medical profession, that it is not possible to equate death itself with cessation of the heartbeat. Quite apart from the elective cardiac arrest of open-heart surgery, spontaneous cardiac arrest followed by successful resuscitation is today a commonplace and although the more sensational accounts of occurrences of this kind still refer to the patient being "dead" until restoration of the heartbeat, the use of the quotation marks usually demonstrates that this word is not to be taken literally, for to most people the one aspect of death that is beyond debate is its irreversibility.

(5) In the majority of cases in which a dying patient passes through the processes leading to the irreversible state we call death, successive organic failures eventually reach a point at which brain death occurs and this is the point of no return.

(6) In a minority of cases brain death does not occur as a result of the failure of other organs or systems but as a direct result of severe damage to the brain itself from, perhaps, head injury or spontaneous intracranial haemorrhage. Here the order of events is reversed: instead of failure of such vital functions as heartbeat and respiration eventually resulting in brain death, brain death results in the cessation of spontaneous respiration; this is normally followed within minutes by cardiac arrest due to hypoxia. If, however, oxygenation is maintained by artificial ventilation the heartbeat can continue for some days, and haemoperfusion will for a time be adequate to maintain function in other organs, such as the liver and kidneys.

(7) Whatever the mode of its production, brain death represents the stage at which a patient becomes truly dead, because by then all functions of the brain have permanently and irreversibly ceased. It is not difficult or illogical in any way to equate this with the concept in many religions of the departure of the spirit from the body.

(8) In the majority of cases, since brain death is part of the culmination of a failure of all vital functions, there is no necessity for a doctor specifically to identify brain death individually before

concluding that the patient is dead. In a minority of cases in which it is brain death that causes failure of other organs and systems, the fact that these systems can be artificially maintained even after brain death has made it important to establish a diagnostic routine which will identify with certainty the existence of brain death.

Conclusions

(9) It is the conclusion of the conference that the identification of brain death means that the patient is dead, whether or not the function of some organs, such as a heartbeat, is still maintained by artificial means.

References

1. Conference of Medical Royal Colleges and their Faculties (UK), *BMJ*, 2, (1976): 1187. Reprinted by permission.

2. Conference of Medical Royal Colleges and their Faculties (UK), *Lancet*, 2, (1976): 1069.

Appendix C

Guidelines for the Diagnosis of Brain Death

Canadian Neurocritical Care Group*

Can J Neurol Sci, 26: (1999): 64-66

Brain death is defined as the irreversible loss of the capacity for consciousness combined with the irreversible loss of all brainstem functions including the capacity to breathe.[1,2] Brain death is equivalent to death of the individual, even though the heart continues to beat and spinal cord functions may persist.[1-3]

Guidelines for organ transplantation and the removal of organs from brain-dead donors is a separate issue that is not addressed in this document. Such procedures must respect provincial and institutional guidelines. As a general rule, those individuals who assess patients for brain death should not be part of the transplant team.

Brain death must be determined clinically by an experienced physician and in accord with the accepted medical standards.[1] Thus the guidelines described below are recommendations based on current medical information and experience. As knowledge advances, it can be anticipated that further revisions will be necessary. Because of the major consequences of the diagnosis of brain death, consultation with other physicians experienced in the relevant clinical examinations and diagnostic procedures is usually advisable.

Brain death can usually be diagnosed reliably by clinical criteria alone. However, there are special circumstances when these are not suitable and cannot be applied. These are discussed below under "Special Circumstances" and "Laboratory Tests".

Guidelines

1. An etiology has been established that is capable of causing brain death and potentially reversible causes have been excluded (see Comment 2 below).
2. The patient is in deep coma and shows no response within cranial nerve distribution to stimulation of any part of the body. No movements such as cerebral seizures, dyskinetic movements, decorticate or decerebrate movements arising from the brain should be present (see 1a below).
3. Brainstem reflexes are absent (see 1b below).
4. The patient is apneic when taken off the respirator for an appropriate time (see 1c below.)
5. The conditions listed above persist when the patient is reassessed after a suitable interval (see 2 below).
6. There should be no confounding factors for the application of clinical criteria (see 1c, 2 and Special Circumstances below).

Comments

1. Cessation of brain function
The clinical absence of brain function is defined as the profound coma, apnea and the absence of brainstem reflexes.

a) **Coma**
The patient should be observed for spontaneous behavior and response to noxious stimuli. In particular, there should be no motor response within cranial nerve distribution to stimuli applied to any body regions. There should be no spontaneous or elicited movements (dyskinesias, decorticate or decerebrate posturing or epileptic seizures arising from the brain). However, various spinal reflexes may persist in brain death.

b) **Brain-stem reflexes**
Pupillary light, corneal, vestibulo-ocular and pharyngeal reflexes must be absent. The pupils should be midsize or larger and must be unreactive to light. Care should be taken that atropine or

related drugs that could block the pupillary light reflex have not been given to the patient. The vestibulo-ocular reflexes should be tested with caloric stimulation while the head is 30° above the horizontal. In adults a minimum of 50 ml of ice water should be used. A minimum of 5 minutes should be allowed between testing on each side. Grimacing or other motor response to corneal stimulation or pharyngeal or tracheal suctioning is incompatible with brain death.[1, 4]

c) **Apnea**
Apnea testing requires the availability of blood gas measurement. It is recommended that a **$PaCO_2$** of 60 mm Hg be achieved to ensure that an adequate stimulus is presented to the respiratory center.[5] It is also suggested that the arterial or capillary blood should be acidemic (pH < 7.28) by the end of the apnea test. The following prerequisites are recommended: i) core temperature should be at least 32.2°C, preferably > 36.5°C, to allow an adequate rate of rise of $PaCO_2$. (Great caution must be exercised in patients with subnormal body temperatures. Further, in chronic retainers of carbon dioxide, the apnea test may not be valid.); ii) systolic blood pressure should be 90 mm Hg in adults and within normal limits for age in infants and children; iii) the patient should be euvolemic; iv) an initially normal $PaCO_2$ before apnea testing is begun (40 ± 5 mm Hg); v) pre-oxygenation with 100 oxygen allowing a PaO_2 > 200 mm Hg. In performing the apnea test, it is suggested that 100% oxygen is delivered via a cannula placed in the trachea, or at the level of the carina, while the ventilator is stopped. The arterial PaO_2, $PaCO_2$ and pH should be checked at 8-10 minutes. The apnea test is positive if no respirations are observed over the 8-10 minutes of observation, provided that the $PaCO_2$ rises to greater than 60 mm Hg.[1,3,6]

2. Irreversibility
Cessation of brain function is determined to be irreversible when: the proximate cause of the coma is known and is capable of causing neuronal death; the loss of brainstem function is total and constant over time; reversible causes of brain dysfunction have been excluded. Drug intoxication (particularly barbiturates, sedatives

and hypnotics), treatable metabolic disorders, hypothermia (temperature less than 32.2°C), shock and peripheral nerve or muscle dysfunction due to disease or neuromuscular blocking agents must be excluded. Neuro-imaging, in selected cases, may be useful in documenting a structural cause and determining the extent of anatomical damage.

Re-evaluation is essential to ensure that the nonfunctioning state of the brain is persistent and to reduce the possibility of error. Depending on the etiology, the interval between such examinations may be as short as 2 hours or as long as 24 hours; observation for 24 hours is usually recommended to confirm brain death due to anoxic-ischemic insults (e.g., post-cardiac arrest). In situations where brain death is declared for purposes of organ transplantation, local regulations may stipulate specific intervals for reassessment.

Special Circumstances

Neonates and young children

In children with a conceptional age of 52 weeks or older (more than 2 months post-term) the adult clinical criteria can be applied. Clinical criteria alone are not sufficient in the determination of brain death in infants under this age.[7-9] The basic tenets accepted in adults that apply to children include: (i) the importance of excluding remediable or reversible conditions, specially toxic and metabolic derangement and the effects of sedative drugs, paralytic agents, hypothermia and hypotension, (ii) physical examination criteria must be satisfied (outlined under "comments" above) and (iii) irreversibility must be ensured by re-evaluation at specified intervals. It is recommended that: (a) for term newborns (greater than 38 weeks gestation) and young infants, aged 7 days to 2 months, that the clinical examination and a radionuclide brain flow study be done, (b) for those 2 months to 1 year, two examinations and EEGs separated by at least 24 hours was suggested; a repeat examination and EEG would not be necessary if a concomitant radionuclide angiographic study failed to visualize cerebral arteries, and (c) in those over 1 year of age, an observation period of at least 12 hours is recommended. However, in those comatose due to hypoxic-ischemic encephalopathy, at least 24 hours of observation is suggested. The validity of the application of clinical criteria to preterm infants is still uncertain. Further guidelines are needed. Clearly additional supportive investigative tests, e.g., those of brain perfusion, are needed to substantiate the diagnosis of brain death in this group.

Inability To Apply The Clinical Criteria

Some clinical situations may preclude the valid application of the listed clinical criteria, e.g., trauma to the eyes, middle or inner ear injuries, cranial neuropathies, severe pulmonary disease and some cases of profound metabolic and endocrine disturbances. In these situations, the most reliable means of determining brain death is the demonstration of the absence of brain perfusion. Some conditions may mimic brain death, e.g., hypothermia, drug intoxication, the use of neuromuscular blocking and anticholinergic agents and shock. These should be excluded or reversed before applying the clinical criteria. In some situations, the use of reliable laboratory tests for brain perfusion, providing the blood pressure is normal, are utilized to confirm the diagnosis of brain death.

Laboratory Tests

Although brain death can be established reliably by clinical criteria alone, special tests can be used to support the clinical diagnosis. These are discussed below.

Cerebral angiography

A selective 4-vessel angiogram is done with the iodinated contrast medium injected under high pressure in both the anterior and posterior circulations. It should be assured that the mean arterial pressure is at least 80 mm Hg. In brain death no intracranial perfusion other than an occasional filling of the superior sagittal sinus is seen. The lack of intracranial perfusion other than filling of the superior sagittal sinus is strongly confirmatory of brain death.[10, 11]

Radionuclide scanning

This is being increasingly used as an alternative to cerebral angiography as a test of cerebral perfusion. Two-planar imaging using a radioactively-labeled substance that readily crosses the blood-brain barrier (such as Technetium-99m hexamthylproplyeneamine oxme [^{99m}Tc-HMPAO] is recommended.[12] In brain death no uptake is seen in the brain parenchyma. Alternatively, the rapid bolus injection of serum albumin labeled with Technetium-99m is given, followed by imaging with a gamma camera. In brain death there is lack of penetration of ^{99m}Tc-HMPAO into the brain parenchyma or no intracranial perfusion seen in the arterial phase following the bolus injection of radio-labeled albumin. Late filling of the superior sagittal sinus may occur, however.

Transcranial Doppler ultrasonography

Using a 2 MHz pulsed Doppler instrument, the intracranial arteries are insonated bilaterally, including the middle and/or anterior cerebral arteries and the vertebral or basilar artery.[13] The finding of absent diastolic or reverberating flow or small systolic peaks have been reported in brain death. The absence of transcranial Doppler signals cannot be taken as evidence of brain death, as 10% of people do not have temporal insonation windows.[5] The test should be performed and interpreted by qualified individuals with considerable experience.

Other imaging tests

Although magnetic resonance imaging (MRI) techniques hold promise, they have not been sufficiently studied or validated to be used as the sole confirmatory test at this time. Neuro-imaging, e.g., with MRI or computed axial tomography, may help to confirm the structural nature and extent of damage in selected cases.

Electroneurophysiological tests

The electroencephalogram (EEG) is of some confirmatory value and may have a place in selecting certain individuals, e.g., very young children, for apnea testing. The EEG does not, however, adequately assess brainstem function and should not be used as the sole confirmatory test for brain death. The use of evoked potentials, including **brainstem auditory and somatosensory evoked potential testing**, has promise, but these have not been sufficiently validated. Furthermore, they are highly dependent on technical quality and require considerable expertise and experience for reliable performance and interpretation.

Atropine test

The absence of an increase in heart rate after the intravenous injection of 2 mg of atropine, is confirmatory of the absence of vagal tone and is helpful in confirming dysfunction of the caudal brainstem.[14, 15] Although helpful, the atropine test is not sufficient as the sole confirmatory test of brain death. Because of the anticholinergic effects on pupillary reactivity and EEG, the test should be performed after completion of clinical and electroencephalographic testing. Further, the test is not valid in cases of autonomic neuropathy or following cardiac transplantation with denervation of the autonomic fibres to the heart.

These guidelines were prepared by a subcommittee of the Canadian Neurocritical Care Group at the request of the Canadian Neurological Society, the Canadian Neurosurgical Society, the Canadian Association of Child Neurology and the Canadian Society of Clinical Neurophysiologists.

*Members of Canadian Neurocritical Care Group: Drs. Marc-André Beaulieu, Shashikant Seshia, Jeanne Teitelbaum and Bryan Young, *Can J Neurol Sci*, 26: (1999): 64-66.

References

1. Brain Death Task Force: Guidelines for the diagnosis of brain death, *CMAJ*, 136: (1987): 200A-200B.

2. Working Group of Conference of Medical Colleges and their Faculties in the United Kingdom: Criteria for the diagnosis of brainstem death. *JR Coll Phys (London)*, 29, (1995): 281-282.

3. Medical Consultants on the Diagnosis of Death to the President's Commission: Guidelines for the determination of death, *JAMA*, 246, (1981): 2184-2185.

4. Pallis, C., Harley, D. H., *ABC of Brainstem Death*, 2nd edn., (London: British Medical Journal Publishing Group, 1996).

5. Wijdicks, E. F. M., Determining brain death in adults, *Neurology*, 45, (1995): 1003-1011.

6. Quality Standards Subcommittee of the American Academy of Neurology: Practice parameters for determining brain death in adults, *Neurology*, 45, (1995): 1012-1014.

7. Task Force for the Determination of Brain Death in Children: Guidelines for the determination of brain death in children, *Arch Neurol*, 44, (1998): 587-588.

8. Okamoto, K., Sugimoto, T., Return of spontaneous respiration in an infant who fulfilled current criteria to determine brain death, *Pediatrics*, 96, (1995): 518-520.

9. Fishman, M. A., Validity of brain death in infants, *Pediatrics*, 96, (1995): 513-515.

10. Bradac, G. B., Simon, R. S., Angiography in brain death, *Neuroradiology*, 7, (1974): 25-28.

11. Albertini, A., Schonfeld, S., Hiatt, M., Hegyi, T., Digital subtraction angiography: A new approach to brain death determination in the newborn, *Pediatr Radiol*, 23, (1993): 195-197.

12. Yatim, A., Mercatello, A., Coronel, B., et al., 99mTc-HMPAO cerebral scintigraphy in the diagnosis of brain death, *Transplant Proc*, 23, (1991): 2491.

13. Ropper, A. H., Kehne, S. M., Weschler, L., Transcranial Doppler in brain death, *Neurology*, 37, (1987): 1733-1735.

14. Drory, Y., Ouaknine, G., Kosary, I. Z., Kellermann, J. J., Electrocardiographic findings in brain death: description and presumed mechanism, *Chest*, 67, (1975): 425-432.

15. Ouaknine, G. E., Mercier, C., La valeur du test à l'atropine dans la confirmation de la mort cérébrale, *Union Med Can*, 114, (1985): 76-80.

Reprinted by permission from the *Canadian Journal of Neurological Sciences*.

Appendix D

Uniform Determination of Death Act, USA

This Act provides comprehensive bases for determining death in all situations. It is based on a ten-year evolution of statutory language on this subject. The first statute passed in Kansas in 1970. In 1972, Professor Alexander Capron and Dr. Leon Kass refined the concept further in "A Statutory Definition of the Standards for Determining Human Death: An Appraisal and a Proposal," 121 Pa. L. Rev. 87. In 1975, the Law and Medicine Committee of the American Bar Association (ABA) drafted a Model Definition of Death Act. In 1978, the National Conference of Commissioners on Uniform State Laws (NCCUSL) completed the Uniform Brain Death Act. It was based on the prior work of the ABA. In 1979, the American Medical Association (AMA) created its own Model Determination of Death statute. In the meantime, some twenty-five state legislatures adopted statutes based on one or another of the existing models.

The interest in these statutes arises from modern advances in lifesaving technology. A person may be artificially supported for respiration and circulation after all brain functions cease irreversibly. The medical profession, also, has developed techniques for determining loss of brain functions while cardiorespiratory support is administered. At the same time, the common law definition of death cannot assure recognition of these techniques. The common law standard for determining death is the cessation of all vital functions, traditionally demonstrated by "an absence of spontaneous respiratory and cardiac functions." There is, then, a potential disparity between current and accepted biomedical practice and the common law.

The proliferation of model acts and uniform acts, while indicating a legislative need, also may be confusing. All existing acts have the same principal goal–extension of the common law to include the new techniques for determination of death. With no essential disagreement on policy, the associations which have drafted statutes met to find common language. This Act contains that common language, and is the result of agreement between the ABA, AMA, and NCCUSL.

Part (1) codifies the existing common law basis for determining death—total failure of the cardiorespiratory system. Part (2) extends the common law to include the new procedures for determination of death based upon irreversible loss of all brain functions. The overwhelming majority of cases will continue to be determined according to part (1). When artificial means of support preclude a determination under part (1), the Act recognizes that death can be determined by the alternative procedures.

Under part (2), the entire brain must cease to function, irreversibly. The "entire brain" includes the brainstem, as well as the neocortex. The concept of "entire brain" distinguishes determination of death under this Act from "neocortical death" or "persistent vegetative state." These are not deemed valid medical or legal bases for determining death.

This Act also does not concern itself with living wills, death with dignity, euthanasia, rules on death certificates, maintaining life support beyond brain death in cases of pregnant women or of organ donors, and protection for the dead body. These subjects are left to other law.

This Act is silent on acceptable diagnostic tests and medical procedures. It sets the general legal standard for determining death, but not the medical criteria for doing so. The medical profession remains free to formulate acceptable medical practices and to utilize new biomedical knowledge, diagnostic tests, and equipment.

It is unnecessary for the Act to address specifically the liability of persons who make determinations. No person authorized by law to determine death, who makes such a determination in accordance with the Act, should, or will be, liable for damages in any civil action or subject to prosecution in any criminal proceeding for his acts or the acts of others based on that determination. No person who acts in good faith, in reliance on a determination of death, should, or will be, liable for damages in any civil action or subject to prosecution in any criminal proceeding for his acts. There is no need to deal with these issues in the text of this Act.

Time of death, also, is not specifically addressed. In those instances in which time of death affects legal rights, this Act states the bases for determining death. Time of death is a fact to be determined with all others in each individual case, and may be resolved, when in doubt, upon expert testimony before the appropriate court.

Finally, since this Act should apply to all situations, it should not be joined with the Uniform Anatomical Gift Act so that its application is limited to cases of organ donation.

UNIFORM DETERMINATION OF DEATH ACT

Section

1 . Determination of Death.

2. Uniformity of Construction and Application.

3. Short Title.

Be it enacted . . .

§ 1. [Determination of Death]. An individual who has sustained either (1) irreversible cessation of circulatory and respiratory functions, or (2) irreversible cessation of all functions of the entire brain, including the brain stem, is dead. A determination of death must be made in accordance with accepted medical standards.

§ 2. [Uniformity of Construction and Application]. This Act shall be applied and construed to effectuate its general purpose to make uniform the law with respect to the subject of this Act among states enacting it.

§ 3. [Short Title]. This Act may be cited as the Uniform Determination of Death Act.

Appendix E

Euthanasia and assisted suicide (update 1998)

This policy replaces a previous policy entitled *Physician-Assisted Death 1995*.

The CMA does not support euthanasia and assisted suicide. It urges its members to uphold the principles of palliative care. The following policy summary includes definitions of euthanasia and assisted suicide, background information, basic ethical principles and physician concerns about legalization of euthanasia and assisted suicide.

Definitions

The CMA defines euthanasia and assistance in suicide as follows.

Euthanasia means knowingly and intentionally performing an act that is explicitly intended to end another person's life and that includes the following elements: the subject is a competent, informed person with an incurable illness who has voluntarily asked for his or her life to be ended; the agent knows about the person's condition and desire to die, and commits the act with the primary intention of ending the life of that person; and the act is undertaken with empathy and compassion and without personal gain.

Assistance in suicide means knowingly and intentionally providing a person with the knowledge or means or both required to commit suicide, including counseling about lethal doses of drugs, prescribing such lethal doses or supplying the drugs.

Euthanasia and assisted suicide are often regarded as morally equivalent, although there is a clear practical distinction, as well as a legal distinction, between them.

Euthanasia and assisted suicide, as understood here, must be distinguished from the withholding or withdrawal of inappropriate, futile or unwanted medical treatment or the provision of compassionate palliative care, even when these practices shorten life.

Background

Euthanasia and assisted suicide are opposed by almost every national medical association and prohibited by the law codes of almost all countries. A change in the legal status of these practices in Canada would represent a major shift in social values and behaviour. For the medical profession to support such a change and subsequently participate in these practices, a fundamental reconsideration of traditional medical ethics would be required.

Physicians, other health professionals, academics, interest groups, the media, legislators and the judiciary are all deeply divided about the advisability of changing the current legal prohibition of euthanasia and assisted suicide. Because of the controversial nature of these practices, their undeniable importance to physicians and their unpredictable effects on the practice of medicine, these issues must be approached cautiously and deliberately by the profession and society.

Basic ethical principles

Although euthanasia and assisted suicide are not mentioned explicitly in the CMA Code of Ethics, the code has traditionally been interpreted as opposing these practices. The following articles of the code are relevant to CMA policy on this issue.

1. "Consider first the well-being of the patient." This means that the care of patients, in this case those who are terminally ill or who face an indefinite life span of suffering or meaninglessness, must be physicians' first consideration.

2. "Provide for appropriate care for your patient, including

physical comfort and spiritual and psychosocial support, even when cure is no longer possible."

3. "Provide your patients with the information they need to make informed decisions about their medical care, and answer their questions to the best of your ability."

4. "Respect the right of a competent patient to accept or reject any medical care recommended."

5. "Ascertain wherever possible and recognize your patient's wishes about the initiation, continuation or cessation of life-sustaining treatment."

6. "Accept a share of the profession's responsibility to society in matters relating to . . . legislation affecting the health or well-being of the community . . ."

7. "Inform your patient when your personal morality would influence the recommendation or practice of any medical procedure that the patient needs or wants."

These principles cannot, by themselves, determine whether euthanasia and assisted suicide should be permitted. Nevertheless, they are relevant to the debate. The first five emphasize the importance of patient well-being and autonomy, the sixth balances this with responsibility to society, and the seventh defends physician autonomy if the law were to be changed.

CMA policy on physician participation in euthanasia and assisted suicide

Canadian physicians should not participate in euthanasia and assisted suicide.

Physician concerns about legalization of euthanasia and assisted suicide

The CMA recognizes that it is the prerogative of society to decide whether the laws dealing with euthanasia and assisted suicide should be changed. The CMA wishes to contribute the perspective of the medical profession to the examination of the legal, social and ethical issues.

Before any change in the legal status of euthanasia or assisted suicide is considered, the CMA urges that the following concerns be addressed.

1. Adequate palliative-care services must be made available to all Canadians. The 1994 CMA General Council unanimously approved a motion that Canadian physicians should uphold the principles of palliative care.

The public has clearly demonstrated its concern with our care of the dying. The provision of palliative care for all who are in need is a mandatory precondition to the contemplation of permissive legislative change. Euthanasia and assisted suicide should never be chosen by patients because of concerns about the availability of palliative care. Efforts to broaden the availability of palliative care in Canada should be intensified.

2. Suicide-prevention programs should be maintained and strengthened where necessary. Although attempted suicide is not illegal, it is often the result of temporary depression or unhappiness. Society rightly supports efforts to prevent suicide, and physicians are expected to provide life-support measures to people who have attempted suicide. In any debate about providing assistance in suicide to relieve the suffering of persons with incurable diseases, the interests of those at risk of attempting suicide for other reasons must be safeguarded.

3. A Canadian study of medical decision making during dying should be undertaken. We know relatively little about the frequency of various medical decisions made near the end of life, how these decisions are made and the satisfaction of patients,

families, physicians and other caregivers with the decision-making process and outcomes. Physicians are involved in making decisions concerning whether to withhold or withdraw treatment and whether to administer sedatives and analgesics in doses that may shorten life. It is alleged that some physicians are providing euthanasia or assistance in suicide. Hence, a study of medical decision making during dying is needed to evaluate the current state of Canadian practice. This evaluation would help determine the possible need for change and identify what those changes should be. If physicians participating in such a study were offered immunity from prosecution based on information collected, as was done during the Remmelink commission in the Netherlands, the study could substantiate or refute the repeated allegations that euthanasia and assisted suicide take place.

4. The public should be given adequate opportunity to comment on any proposed change in legislation.

5. Consideration should be given to whether any proposed legislation can restrict euthanasia and assisted suicide to the indications intended. If euthanasia or assisted suicide or both are permitted for competent, suffering, terminally ill patients, there may be legal challenges, based on the Canadian Charter of Rights and Freedoms, to extend these practices to others who are not competent, suffering or terminally ill. Such extension is the "slippery slope" that many fear. Courts may be asked to hear cases involving euthanasia for incompetent patients on the basis of advance directives or requests from proxy decision makers. Such cases could involve neurologically impaired patients or newborns with severe congenital abnormalities. Psychiatrists recognize the possibility that a rational, otherwise well person may request suicide. Such a person could petition the courts for physician-assisted suicide.

Is there a way to consider these possibilities in advance, so that the law is determined by the wishes of society, as expressed through Parliament, rather than by court decisions?

Conclusion

This statement has been developed to help physicians, the public and politicians participate in any re-examination of the current legal prohibition of euthanasia and assisted suicide and arrive at a solution in the best interests of Canadians.

Pari Publishing is an independent publishing company, based in a medieval Italian village. Our books appeal to a broad readership and focus on innovative ideas and approaches from new and established authors who are experts in their fields. We publish books in the areas of science, society, psychology, and the arts.

Our books are available at all good bookstores or online at
www.paripublishing.com

If you would like to add your name to our email list to receive information about our forthcoming titles and our online newsletter please contact us at **newsletter@paripublishing.com**

Visit us at **www.paripublishing.com**

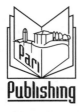

Pari Publishing Sas
Via Tozzi, 7
58040 Pari (GR)
Italy

Email: info@paripublishing.com